12/20

GRIT & GRACE

GRIT & GRACE

TRAIN THE MIND
TRAIN THE BODY
OWN YOUR LIFE

TIM MCGRAW
WITH AMELY GREEVEN

THORNDIKE PRESS
A part of Gale, a Cengage Company

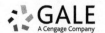

Copyright © 2019 by Project #268866, Inc.

Additional photography by Thien Phan and Becky Fluke.

ALL RIGHTS RESERVED

Thorndike Press® Large Print Nonfiction.

The text of this Large Print edition is unabridged.

Other aspects of the book may vary from the original edition.

Set in 16 pt. Plantin.

**LIBRARY OF CONGRESS CIP DATA ON FILE.
CATALOGUING IN PUBLICATION FOR THIS BOOK
IS AVAILABLE FROM THE LIBRARY OF CONGRESS**

ISBN-13: 978-1-4328-8108-5 (hardcover alk. paper)

Published in 2020 by arrangement with Harper Wave, an imprint of HarperCollins Publishers

Printed in Mexico

Print Number: 01   Print Year: 2020

CONTENTS

5

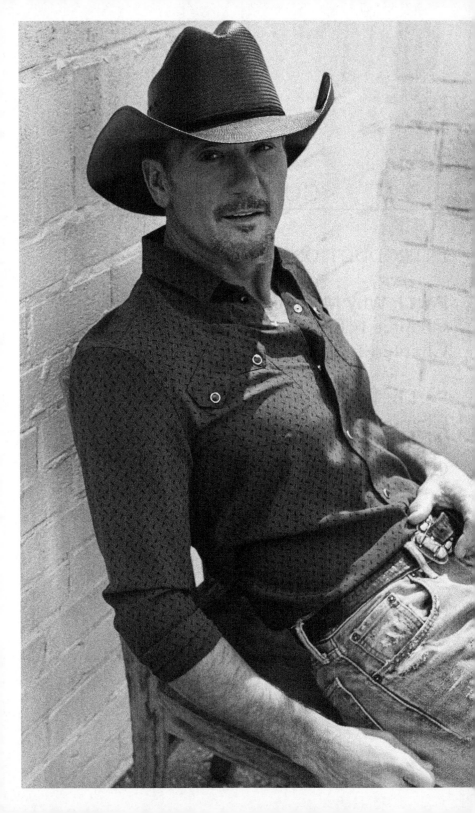

INTRODUCTION

Kansas City, Missouri: In the predawn light, a convoy of tour buses and tractor trailers park in a row at the Sprint Arena, where later that night I'll take the stage with my band. Setting down coffees and sleepily rolling open the doors, the crew starts to unload and organize the kind of gear that a large-scale musical tour production requires: tiers of sound equipment, walls of video monitors, cases of instruments, racks of wardrobe, and catering for a small army.

Except for one of them: the trailer with "TRUMAV" emblazoned on the side. Unlike the others, it didn't travel 500 miles through the night from last night's show to bring electronics for the stage and set. Instead, it parks in the very back parking lot, next to my tour bus. And when the guys roll open its doors, there's no sonic equipment in sight except for an old stereo and a couple of small speakers. Instead, it's stocked with stuff that takes extra muscle to move: fifty-foot battle ropes for fierce full-body conditioning; giant tires for flipping, sledgehammers for pounding, and a cluster of rowing machines, kettlebells, and barbells, all intended to push our bodies and minds to the edge.

Welcome to what my longtime fiddle player Deano fondly calls the Gorilla Yard — our functional fitness playground filled with things to throw, pound, lift, and pull. It's part garage gym on overdrive, part Ninja Warrior obstacle course, and part town-square gathering spot. It's where my band and crew and I sweat together, leave our frustrations on the asphalt, and get all cylinders firing so we can bring the best we've got to the audience waiting on the other side of the stage. It's about as far away from my former pregame rituals as I could imagine — kicking back with a cold one or two in order put a blur on any jitters. One thing's for sure: my band and I don't roll into town the way we used to.

Now, instead of dulling our senses, we're heightening them. There's a kind of peacefulness that settles into you after a great workout; your body has built up tension, then released it, and a flush of clarity and wakefulness moves through you even if your muscles burn and shake. Spending energy has actually *given* you energy — and if you take a minute to notice it, you realize you're feeling every part of yourself more acutely. You're finding aliveness in every nook and cranny, as if someone just turned up the lights.

Come 8:00 p.m., the first notes of the night play and I grab my hat, ready to fire things up. I feel a whole lot better at fifty-one than I did ten years ago, when I was at a respectable height professionally but operating more than a few levels shy of my personal best. I'm more energized and stronger physically, and I'm stronger mentally, too. Who knows if the audience feels the difference, but *I* feel the difference, and I credit it to a single decision I made just over ten years ago. That one, seemingly small, but life-changing decision was to move my body every day so I could take ownership of my health.

I came to it like a lot of us come to turning points: By touching a place I don't care to go back to — a dark place where I felt like a lot of my life was out of my control. Maybe I had to make contact with that bottom in order to push back to the surface, determined to turn things around before my luck ran out and a slide became a crash. It wasn't comfortable, and I'm not always proud of the ways I behaved, obscured as I was back then in a mix of denial and neglect, but it launched a journey of trimming the fat in every area of life and carving away the excess to get to a better version of myself. Today my body is leaner, my mind is clearer, my sense of purpose is sharper, and my relationships are deeper. Health might start in the body, but it extends way beyond the physical; it's about your connections to the world and people around you, and your ability to serve and give. The decade since I chose to once and for all take ownership of my health has taught me that lesson most of all.

This book is about what happened when I made that one small choice and how it led me from a low point to the better path I'm on today. It didn't happen overnight and it certainly involved a few mistakes along the way, but it schooled me in three important lessons:

1 One small choice to move your body daily can spark a cascade of changes that will turn around the health of your body and mind.

2 It's never too late to start, and, if you commit with purpose and push

a little more than you might normally push, even small efforts count big. A journey can start with just a few degrees of change. Keep at it, and over time that few-degree deviation will lead you to a whole new place.

3 Transforming your health is not just about knowing what to do. It's about knowing why you're doing it, and discovering what stands in the way. Without getting your mental muscles in shape, the road can get rockier than it needs to be and have more stops and starts.

Athleticism and sport have been intertwined into my whole way of being since an early age. It's literally in my DNA. Even so, I lost contact with that part of myself and — foolishly — let the fire dwindle to the point where it almost went out. Life served me a good lesson in humility, and that led me to starting over from close to scratch. I leapt out of a slump at age forty, hit full stride at forty-five, and now at fifty-two it's coming together quite nicely. I didn't follow a playbook or have some guru squad of trainers overseeing every step. I've taken more of a maverick approach: Get a vision of what I want to achieve, go by gut instinct, and figure it out by doing it. I've always thought that if you can just get started, and keep at it, then you're more than halfway to something. You can learn techniques and refine things as you go.

Except that . . . *how do you get started and how do you keep at it once you start?* That's the million-dollar question! If we had it solved, our present crisis in physical and mental health wouldn't be hurting us quite as hard as it is. I'll do my best to share what works for me and what has helped more than a few (willing) recruits from the McGraw music family — all of whom started from different places — take ownership of their health, too. Getting moving in *any* which way is like striking a match or sending a flare into the night. It can help you find a part of yourself that might have been lost in the woods for a while but, I promise, is out there nonetheless: the part of you that wants to feel good. I call this your inner maverick; it's the bigger, better part of you who believes better is *always* possible and that nobody else's experience or opinion of who you are, how you look, or what you can accomplish need apply.

If I've learned anything in my life — finding my way out of small-town Louisiana, dirt poor as a kid and sometimes laughed at for my dreams — it's that the greatest asset we have is feeling that burn to be better. The burn can be frustrating. It can get uncomfortable. It can even get destructive if you don't know how to use it. But heat properly directed can drive change. What I want to share is that there's a lot of energy available inside if you know how to find it, fan it, and keep some oxygen on it. And sometimes it takes another person showing you some in-the-field tricks for catching an ember and turning it into a fire.

Focusing on my physical health hasn't just made my body healthier, it's made me healthier at every level. Moving daily and exercising regularly were pebbles that set off a ripple effect, improving the way I eat, sleep, relate to others, and show up both personally and professionally. It made me a better person to be around. I've been blessed to meet folks before my shows who tell me that seeing me take control of my fitness inspired them to do the same with theirs; something about my journey tilted their axis a little and helped them change course. If even just part of what follows ripples out into your life, I hope it ignites the urge to take a chance like I did and choose one small thing that, if you let it, can change the next thing, then the next thing, until one day you look up and realize you've turned yourself in a new direction.

Though you'll find the mental and physical tools I use to maintain my health in the pages that follow, you certainly don't have to use them exactly as written. Everyone's road looks a little different, and personally rigid rules aren't my thing. I've written the two main sections of the book, Train the Mind and Train the Body, in such a way that — hopefully — you'll find some wisdom you can use whether you've already established a fitness practice and have an activity you love doing, or whether it's been a while and you've been waiting for inspiration to start something new. Even if you do already work out regularly, I've learned from experience that just when you think you have it dialed, you realize how much more there is to discover. That's what makes the path never-ending and always interesting. So keep an open mind, dive in, and let's have some fun!

PART I
WHY MOVEMENT MATTERS

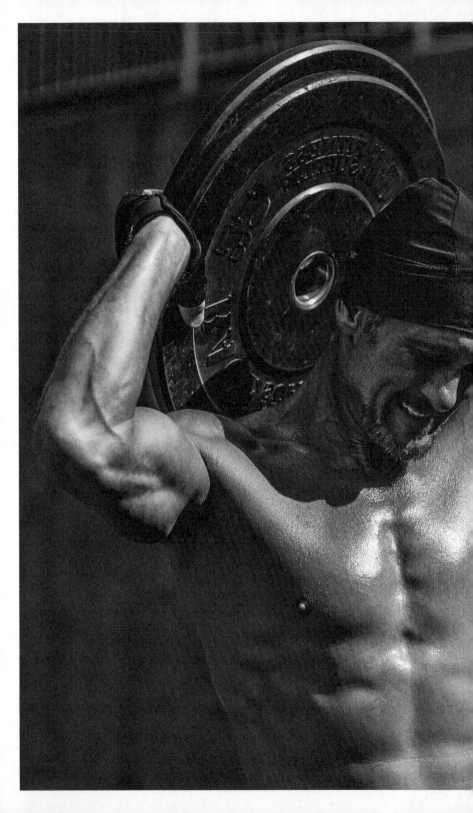

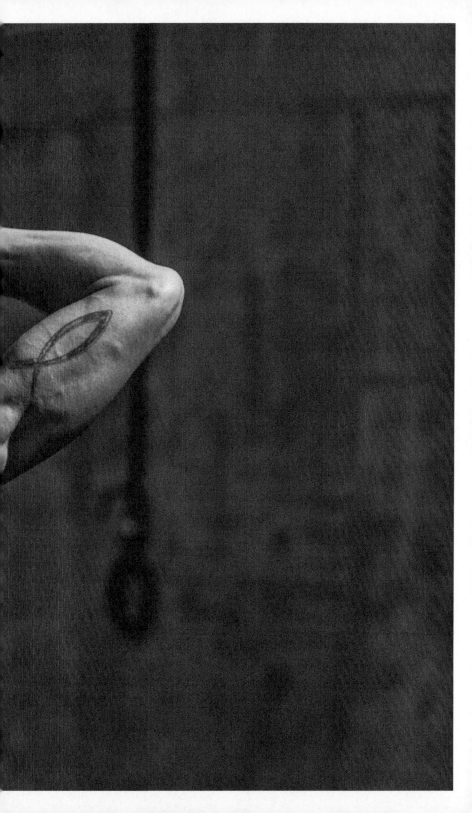

I remember the moment when I clicked into fully owning my health. We were touring in the summertime back in 2011, the nights as hot and sweaty as country music's supposed to be — jeans-and-white-T-shirt kinds of nights where it's all about slinging sweat and having fun. We rolled into Detroit to play at the DTE Energy Music Theater. There's always an incredible crowd for a show like that, and the guys and I were out back of the amphitheater working out harder than usual to get fully primed and as amped as could be. All of a sudden, I had an epiphany. It was like the seas parted and I could see so clearly how the work I'd been doing seriously for the previous two years, staying consistent and honing my discipline, was paying off; the vision I'd been working toward of "best shape of my life" was becoming a reality that I could continue to take further. My body felt good, my mind was clear, and there was a lot less falling off track than in years prior. I saw how the benefits were rippling out into my career and my home life, and I could see where I was headed. I understood how no matter what unfortunate events, mistakes, or embarrassments had happened prior to that moment, I had the complete right to good health and I could claim it if I worked for it. This realization came with a counter-check: It was also overwhelmingly clear that nobody could give that good health *away* but me.

Taking ownership is the first step in creating a different kind of relationship with yourself. Ownership means taking responsibility for your health and being fully invested in building a better version of yourself. When I say "invested" I don't mean financially, because developing fitness doesn't have to cost you if you don't have much to spend. I'm referring to an investment that is mental and spiritual as well as physical. You buy in with your mind by aligning your thoughts with your goals, developing discipline, and embracing routine and structure. You buy in with your spirit by having trust, faith, and hope in the process. And you buy in with your body by putting in the work, by starting strong and finishing stronger each time.

Ownership isn't a flash-in-the-pan

resolution that burns bright then goes out. It's not a thirty-day cleanse or transformation. Ownership means you've bought in fully for the long haul. It's like owning a home rather than renting. You sink some resources into keeping it well cared for, shore up any leaks and holes, and repair the foundations and infrastructure if it needs it, knowing that doing the hard work now will prevent depreciation over time. And because you've invested time and effort, when you have a bad day or you're in a bad mood, you don't just give up on a whim. In that regard, I guess you could say it's like a ride-or-die relationship with your best friend. Or a marriage. Actually, both of these comparisons are pretty apt, because on this journey you become your own soul mate.

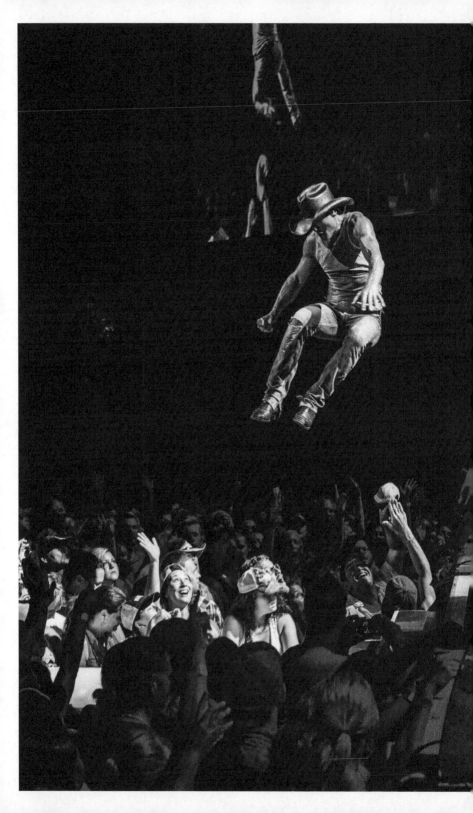

CHAPTER 1

FROM LOSING IT
TO OWNING IT

I had never done anything so wild during a show before. I'd just crossed to the far right of the stage in the middle of performing "Real Good Man" in front of thirteen thousand people at an amphitheater in Tampa, Florida. My band leader and guitarist, Denny, had met me there for a beat — syncing his movement to arrive at the same spot simultaneously — and then, pivoting on my heel to face forward again, I spied it: the long metal runway that extended from the middle of the stage out into the audience like a big letter "T." The ramp wasn't exactly close by; it lay a good few feet below me and at least twelve feet over to my left, and in between me and it was not only a swathe of airspace, but the heads and raised arms of audience members, swaying to the music, faces turned to the lights. And for some ungodly reason, or maybe some godly inspiration, every cell in my body yelled at me, "Jump!"

I leapt off the step with my left leg out-stretched, like a hurdler taking off for the 400-meter race, arced over the outstretched hands, landed one foot on the metal runway with my ankle, knee, and hip absorbing the impact easily, and then felt my whole back body propelling me into a medal-winning sprint to the end of the runway. A sensation of indescribable liberation shot through me like lightning. I'd seen something big, wanted it badly, and done it all-in, fully trusting my body to pull it off.

Then my brain screamed, "Damn. I *did* that?!" I'd just transgressed my cardinal rule: Never risk busting your ass live on-stage, because you will never live it down.

For a musician, hitting that spot where you can really let it all pour out, performing with-out conscious thought or calculation, comes down to training consistently — practicing and then practicing more so that when it's game night, it feels easy. It also comes down to an X factor, something you can't as eas-ily quantify, but that involves confidence. When you have both, you get to feel free, and that's when the magic happens.

The way I view performing is that when you're in the audience and I'm on the stage, we're in a relationship together. When I walk into that arena through one entrance, and you walk into it through yours, no matter how each of us has been feeling up until that moment, we enter a contract with each other. I agree I'm going to suspend ordinary life for a minute; you agree you're going to suspend ordinary life for a minute, and neither one of us is gonna scrutinize the other too closely. We're going to jump in the stream together, let the energy move us and agree that this is not who I am all day, and this is not who you are all day, and let's both not be those people tonight and just have fun.

And boy is it easier to show up for this relationship when your instrument is tuned up, well calibrated, and comfortable to play. In my case, my instrument is my body. And when it's in peak condition, it feels as if the gates are open. I can step past the me of daily life, let the spirit move me, and together we can connect through music. Those are the shows when we all feel it — we have the time of our lives.

A decade before making that soaring leap, when I was technically the age that, had I been an athlete, I would've had just one or two good years left in me, I would never have attempted such a feat. Let alone stuck the landing.

I was doing well by anyone's standards. My wife, Faith, and I had just come off the top-grossing tour in the history of country music, and I was starting to make some of the most meaningful music of my career. I'd had a few roles in movies on the side and developed some philanthropic endeavors that were making an impact, like Neighbor's Keeper Fund, a charity that Faith and I started to address communities in need or the work for the Tug McGraw Foundation devoted to enhancing the quality of life for those diagnosed with debilitating brain conditions that I helped launch in honor of my dad, Tug. To the outside world, these efforts had been meeting pretty high targets and even sometimes exceeding them. But on the inside, I had been letting things slip gradually — first a little, and then a little more, until it eventually added up to a lot.

I was forty pounds heavier than I should have been; had considerably more body fat than my frame wanted on it and a lot less muscle than I have today. My energy levels, which have always been high, even borderline off-the-charts, were unpredictable, dipping at times to sluggish levels of fatigue. My immune system was struggling to keep up with my lifestyle and I was getting sick too often. And my mind was muddled, its bandwidth crowded with more anxious thoughts than normal. That made me quick to tip into reactivity and stress. My mind races at 90 mph on a good day — it can be a little manic in there, but it's how I'm wired. I've come to accept my brain's restless motion as the source of my best ideas — the driver of my creativity and my art. But walking it can be a high-wire act because worry, doubt, and anxiety can move along it equally fast, and if I'm out of balance these thoughts can eclipse the others, clouding my outlook and turning it stormy — which is what I was now experiencing.

I hadn't just arrived in this state out of nowhere. The years leading up to turning forty had thrown a few curveballs my way. My father had passed of cancer at the age of fifty-nine, way too soon. Losing a parent at any age will cut you to the core, but when you didn't know your dad growing up and only became close to him as an adult, and when there are still a lot of unresolved feelings about the relationship tangled up in your heart, unexpected loss can put your emotional state into a tailspin. Around the same time, my stepdad died, too; a man who'd occupied a big space in my life as a kid, and not always in the best or most supportive ways. And then my high school coach passed away, adding a further shot to the heart. Coach Butler was one of the only positive male influences I'd had growing up. He saw something special in me and nurtured it through sports. He was tough on me at times — as he should've been — but he always had my best interests in mind, guiding and looking out for me.

When three complex father figures pass during the time when you yourself are being asked to step into a strong father role for your own kids, it can create quite a turmoil inside. Nothing highlights just how little you learned about fathering than having three adolescent daughters who are starting to push you away while profoundly needing you to show up. I'm a pretty tough judge of myself when it comes to just about everything. The fear I might be messing up the most important job I'd been given — fatherhood — shook me to my core. Making things even tougher, the grandmother and grandfather who had been my rocks as a kid passed in the same short span of years. In one clean sweep, five of the elders who'd raised me were gone.

Grief will do funny things to you. It'll make you turn inward to lick your wounds, and if they hurt too much when you look at them, it'll tempt you to dull the soreness with distraction or consumption — anything to make the sorrow recede into a place your senses can't quite detect. I used both those tactics, filling my world with career commitments that made enough noise to drown out the heartache and kept me busy enough to avoid a childhood worth of hurt. That way, in my mind, nobody close to me had to see me sit in a place of vulnerability and pain. And though getting a buzz through drinking was never something I especially liked, it's never too far from hand when you're in the music industry — it's a norm that most everyone agrees on, one color in the paint box of the rock 'n' roll fantasy life. A few beers here and there began helping me be that guy I thought I had to be — the upbeat guy who starts the party and ensures a whole lot of people have a good time. Then there's the other guy I had to be: the leader that keeps a big ship on course, because the unseen side of success in the recording business is that you are running a company, acting as president and CEO. Dozens of people work with you to keep the whole machine working — over a hundred of them when you're on tour — and their livelihoods depend on the artist they work for to hit the ball out of the park again and again. A decade or two ago, a performing artist could afford to have a few off years here and there or make an album or two the public didn't quite get.

Today, the stakes are higher and attention spans are shorter and when your name is on the marquee, there's a lot more pressure to get it right.

In my case, there was another, more contentious layer of challenge: a long-simmering conflict with the record label that, for better or worse, owned my recorded music catalog. For years, they'd been exploiting my contract to dictate when I could and couldn't release new music. As an artist, you always feel you're only as good as your last good song, and to counter that fear, you feel an incredible need for free rein to create and innovate, to take risks and make bold departures. Instead of a working creative collaboration with my label partners, it felt like a dictatorship, and the angst of not holding the reins on my career was excruciating.

The irony is that though you're faced with constant pressure to perform, the lifestyle of a performing artist doesn't exactly lend itself to peak performance. A tour will become a constant party if you let it. You come off a show feeling electrified, and your body, already on an adrenaline high, will make a great case for keeping the feeling going. *Stay up all night! Have that drink and a cheeseburger, you deserve it!* The whole environment can make it easy to get fat and happy fast. And if everyone else is in agreement, you all enable the bad habits to get grooved in deeper, so they become harder and harder to see. Throw in the sleep debt that accumulates, the leaning on caffeine and sugar the next day, plus the travel time and sedentary hours waiting for the show to start, and the very lifestyle that makes it possible to share your spirit with the world can be a ticking time bomb for your body. The added extra-weird twist? Everyone will tell you that you're looking great regardless. The inhabitants of this universe are all wearing rose-colored glasses, and not necessarily in a good way.

My dad, Tug, was a Major League Baseball pitcher. He used to say he never got into the game until the bases were loaded. I'm the same way. I'm the king of the Hail Mary pass; I perform best when the race is down to the wire. If things are too easy, I get bored. (As my managers have pointed out more than a few times, I don't idle well.) There's a rub, a friction, between needing pressure and hating it, and that rub can create great moments. But the flip side is that the pressure can build too high, making everything in life feel urgent, overwhelmingly make-or-break. That can drive a slightly manic person like me to rev too high and start acting like a jerk — or sometimes, it can be completely paralyzing.

Back in this period, I didn't have strategies for living with this duality. I wasn't comfortable sitting back, watching and waiting in stillness. In hindsight, I think it's because if things got quiet, I'd hear the old ghosts that tend to follow at my heels like shadows. The ones that say, *You're just a small-town country singer on a lucky streak — what do you know about success?* Working hard and playing hard kept things noisy enough inside to drown them out. But when you're a partner and a parent, if you don't leave intensity at the door when you come home, it starts to strain the bonds. You don't even realize you're using worldly stresses and pressures as a way to check out of something harder to navigate — like intimacy and being there emotionally for the people who love you most. I know I'm not the only man in the world who worries he isn't showing up for the women in his life like they need. I certainly never saw a healthy role model do it before me. And when men feel inadequate, we tend to pull away further, making the situation even worse.

The strains might have been easier to nip in the bud if I'd had more ability to be present and connect more deeply from the heart.

But I hadn't got there yet. And though music was still my best stress relief, the cocktail of grief and legal drama caused me to retreat inward when I wasn't playing and recording. I drank more to dull the discomfort, and we all know how that goes — you lubricate the wheel that turns you inward to wrestle with your demons or escape them entirely. But doing that makes you feel worse, not better, and the worse you feel, the more the stories in your mind get stronger. *What if you don't have it in you? What if your lucky streak runs out?* It's a vicious cycle.

When the shadows get out from behind your heels and start to gain ground in front of you, it takes a clear mind to see it happening and turn things around. If, like me, you're someone who's not great at dealing with your emotional world, you don't always see it and you may not reach out for help. And if you're the type who does things all-in like I am, you can start to find that the retreat becomes a hole, and a comfortable one at that. Holes are insulating; the noises aren't so loud in there, the lights not so bright, and when people reach in their hands to connect, you can pretend not to see.

The few years after my dad's death became one of the darkest periods of my life.

Then the bill came due.

THE TURNING POINT

When you're maxing out the reserves of your body and not putting anything into the account, eventually your creditors catch up with you. In my case, they came knocking three times.

The first knock happened at Faith's parents' house in Mississippi. We were on a weekend visit when I glimpsed the blood pressure cuff that her mom used to track her health. I was curious; I'd been told a couple of times in physicals that my blood pressure was borderline high but had always shrugged it off a temporary glitch. So I slipped it on. Faith's mom watched the gauge go up and made a yelp. "Holy cow, Tim, that's really high! You need to get checked out!" I choked a little. My own mom had high blood pressure, and I'd probably known on some level it needed watching. But I hadn't realized how lifestyle choices like eating poorly and becoming too sedentary could interact with those genetics and cause it to skyrocket. Having lost my dad before he had a chance to see sixty, the elevated number shook me up. What if I got sick? What would happen to Faith and the girls?

The second knock was to my pride. My daughter Gracie and I had gone out to a Christmas movie near our home in Nashville.

As the trailers played before the show, a scene from a holiday movie in which I had a small part suddenly filled the screen, and with it my face — super-sized and not only because of the thirty-foot screen. "Jeez, Dad," muttered Gracie, not quietly, and making an eye roll in the dark. She didn't have to say another word; the screen said it all. My face was inflated and doughy, and my skin looked tired and dull. It was a punch-in-the-gut moment. I wasn't living in the body I thought I was.

The third knock hit my heart. Faith got tired of me checking out and acting like I had it all handled. I guess I thought I'd fooled my family; I can talk my way around all kinds of trouble and, plus, we'd always made sure not to be apart for more than three days in a row. But there's no fooling four smart southern women. My *emotional* absence was noticed and it was not scoring any points. Very fortunately, I'd married a woman of tremendous strength and clarity. It can't have been easy for Faith to see her life partner making bad choices — especially when those bad choices were starting to hurt our whole family. She has always offered un-conditional love in every situation and never for a second have I doubted her willingness to support whatever step I needed to take to find my way back to health. Yet in that instance, she knew that someone had to lay down the law. Getting real like only she can do, Faith told me, "Partying or family, take your pick." There was no question for me on that answer.

Who knows if Faith's ultimatum would really have borne out, but it scared me enough to think it might. I'd like to say it was the vital stats that had the biggest impact, but frankly it was that damn movie trailer! When your "before" diet picture is blown up several stories high and projected straight at you, I guarantee you won't un-see that in a hurry. The initial shock was aesthetic — the entertainment business can be a cruel judge of regular human failings, and the way it skews things, looking good matters, wrongfully, to an almost *in*human degree. But it was the deeper story the image told that really shook me. Getting heavy hadn't just happened: it had come from drinking carbohydrates, eating easy comfort foods, and letting stress rush through my system without flushing it out through good sleep and exercise. The pounds had packed on as a consequence; my six-foot frame was carrying 215 pounds — three dozen pounds over my fighting weight.

It had just crept up on me — how stupid

had I been? I was like the proverbial frog swimming around in a pot of water growing warmer and warmer, not noticing anything was wrong until the water was at a boil. When I sing, it's with my whole body; my physicality is probably my most valuable asset. I've invested thousands of hours into developing my physical instrument, and this training is what's carried me past seeming obstacles, like the fact that I never studied music or received a formal education in the craft. And just when I was starting to feel like I knew what I was doing and had mastered my craft — I'd dotted all the i's and crossed all the t's in every other aspect of my career — I realized I'd let my health go to hell in a handbasket.

We all get served wake-up calls, even if not in high definition in front of two hundred preteen kids. But mine came in loud and clear. It said, *Tim, you're in a hole. You can keep going this way and risk benching yourself early, or take a look at the hole you're digging, and ask yourself how to get out. Which is it?* I like to think the honest, responsible side of me — and the competitive side of me! — spoke louder. It said, *I have an incredible wife, I have great kids, I want to have grandkids. I have a career I'll throw away if I don't turn this around.* In an instant, the spotlight shone on all the impetuses for change. I wanted to run toward it — and as far away from having Dad Bod as possible.

First things first: Drinking was out. I guess I'm fortunate that, for me, its tentacles weren't that strong. I'd made drinking a crutch, but it didn't have a vise grip, and when I recognized how poorly it was serving my body, my family, and my art, I kicked it to the curb and, frankly, did not look back. Clearer eyed, I assessed the situation. I'd been struggling to hold my center in a world where a lot of things felt out of my control, like loss and death, like the music I'd worked so hard to create, like showing up the way others needed. The smarter, wiser part of myself spoke again: *Control what you can control. Just start there.*

Have you ever had one of those nights when you're lying on your bed after drinking too much and you put one foot on the floor to stop the world spinning? It was kind of like that. I asked, *What's that one foot?*

The answer was *Exercise daily.*

Working out may not be everyone's starting point for turning a bad situation around. There are lots of ways to become the better version of yourself. But movement and athleticism were what I knew best. I've always been an athlete, ever since I was a kid playing

Little League, basketball, and football, and starting years before I knew my real father was a pro baseball player. My happiest times have been spent in motion, moving through space or water or air, feeling the speed, feeling free. I knew from experience how training the body gets your mind in line and helps you rise over walls you could've sworn were insurmountable, and how a good session on the field can brighten a bleak day in thirty minutes. I knew that when you're feeling spun out, the simplest remedy on earth is to work up a sweat and let it all go for a while. But getting my priorities turned around like I had, this part of me had gotten sidelined and neglected, which was tantamount to betrayal.

So I made the choice to commit to the one thing I could control — my body. I would go all in to get that one foot firmly planted on the floor.

The First Six Weeks

I've heard it said that when you're low or lost you can choose to feel lost and do nothing, or feel lost and do something — even though you don't feel like it. Guess which is the choice that people with healthier outcomes take?

It seemed crazy that I identified as an

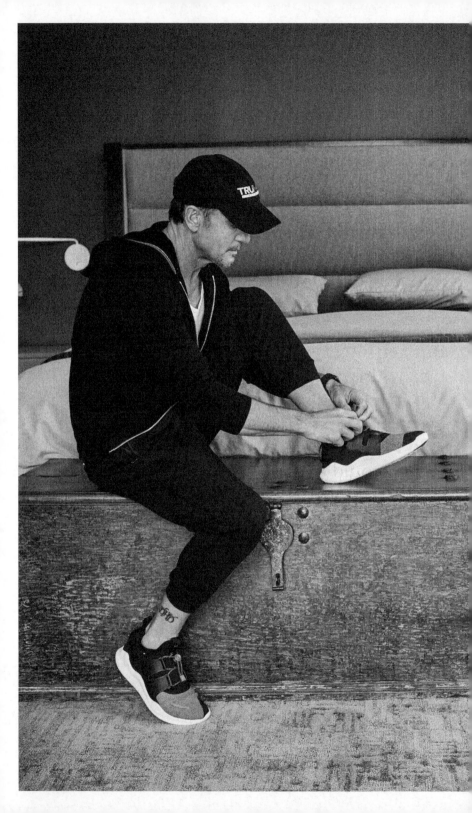

athlete yet had neglected my primary piece of equipment. I'd been cruising on my good genes and natural talent, telling myself they'd carry me through a sedentary spell — without noticing that the spell had become a few seasons. And like many men in their mid-to-late thirties, I still pictured myself as a single man in his twenties — naturally fit, with plenty of time on his hands to play sports and work out at whim. The reality was different; my workouts had become sporadic, or happened in bursts. The hours in the gym weren't adding up to as much as I thought.

So I had two things wrong already, and beneath them, two more. It was a mundane belief that routine is what you do when you give up being passionate, and that being disciplined means being boring.

When you're an artist, it's easy to kid yourself that your best work comes when you let the spirit move you. But that's not actually true. The spirit doesn't always show up if you just hope for it, not work for it — or it might move you in the wrong direction. Like when my band and I were recording our album *Let It Go* in Darkhorse studios outside Nashville. We got the inspiration that indulging in a nightly recording ritual of extra-long Coney Island chili-cheese hot dogs, tater tots, and Dr Pepper would bring good juju — an All American high-fat, high-carb talisman. Really, it was bad habits and messed-up guts that probably caused the cravings. The music would have turned out just as good without it, and our arteries would've been happier.

To meet my goal of exercising daily, I couldn't just wait till I felt like doing it. I needed a structure — something really defined to hang my hat on. So I set a challenge: *Do something physical every single morning for six solid weeks*. I've always thought that if you can do something for six weeks it changes the way you think. After forty-two days straight, new behaviors begin to feel normal. Then you're off and running — so to speak. You put up less resistance because it's just become what you do. Your attitude's gotten an overhaul.

I kept the game plan super simple. To start, I'd walk. In truth, I could have probably hit the gym and lifted weights or done sprints — I wasn't *that* de-conditioned. But I wanted something so close to hand — *Put on shoes. Walk out door* — that no excuse could fly. Growing up in the '70s, we didn't have as many options as we do today; when it was time to train for sports, we just got to the track or court and did what coach said, suicide drills and all. We all knew the formula back then: Show up consistently, put some intention behind the action, and you see results. You get faster, you get stronger, you play better. Today performance experts take that further. They say that in the success equation, effort counts twice as much as talent or skill. My six-week plan was to relearn the science of effort — show up, show up again, and don't question what you're doing every other minute.

Walking is a seriously underrated activity. It's lower impact aerobically, meaning it's not going to radically condition your heart. But it does so much else. As I took my morning walks — sometimes with Faith, sometimes alone; often times on a treadmill but preferably, when home, in nature — I got to feel how walking resets the nervous system. I've learned since that this effect has partly to do with the cross-lateral movements your arms and legs make — opposite leg swinging in rhythm with opposite arm, which stimulates communication between the brain's hemispheres — plus the way you drop into deeper and more regulated breathing, which is the most powerful way to reverse anxiety. It also decompresses the spine, stimulates circulation, and redistributes tension in the body. It literally gets your blood flowing, and along with it a nice hit of oxygen, which energizes your body and mind. What I felt most on those half-hour to hour-long walks was how good it was to rediscover space. With each step and follow-through, step and follow-through, I moved further away from the hole.

After a while I graduated to running. I'd run ten minutes out from a venue where we were performing and ten minutes back, then do some sit-ups and push-ups. The rush of it cleared my head — it felt fantastic. Three of the musicians who'd toured with me longest, my good friends Denny, Dean, and Jeff, were runners who'd done the New York City Marathon. So I jumped on their bandwagon. I couldn't run as long as they could at first, but I was fast. We'd run wherever we were playing that night — through salt mines in Mississippi, around botanical gardens in Sydney. Moving as a pack, soon we were racking back-to-back seven-minute miles. Find your body flying like that, the air blowing cobwebs out of your corners, and you begin to feel back in control.

The six weeks saw my extra weight start to drop off. This wasn't solely from walking and running; those things alone don't tend to cause rapid weight loss. But cutting out the beer that had made me inflamed and bloated had a pretty instantaneous effect. So did gaining the headspace to become more conscious about food because it was the mindless choices toward high-starch meals, made in distraction, and too often made by a truck-stop or take-out kitchen, that had derailed me the most. As the heaviness subsided, I began to feel like myself again. Then the challenge became fun.

One day I was leafing through a fashion magazine that Faith had on the kitchen counter. A black-and-white photo of a chiseled male model with his shirt off, all eight-pack abs and defined deltoids, caught my attention. The guy was probably fifteen, twenty years younger than me and likely had a hotshot trainer helping him look that good. But what flew out of my mouth was, *"Look at that! I'm forty years old, but why can't I do that, too? All it's gonna take is setting my mind to it."* Faith laughed, but she knew me well enough to know that when my mind's set on something, I don't do it half-assed.

Thus started my next level training. I never studied physiology, but I knew that building lean muscle and losing fat isn't rocket science. It's basic physics and biology: Get your body torching enough energy to burn off all the stored sugars and then burn off body fat while giving the muscle tissues enough stress and protein to build themselves stronger. Together, this delivers the strong, lean body that looks defined and (eventually) shredded, but not overly stacked or pumped. Running alone can't achieve this; in fact, running in excess actually breaks down tissues. It has a catabolic effect. I learned this the hard way when my foot got a stress fracture from going too heavy on those seven-minute miles.

Dean, Denny, and I began developing our own kind of strength-building circuit workouts, inspired partly by the classic bodyweight stuff I'd grown up on, partly by the "functional fitness" CrossFit WODS (workouts of the day) that were taking off at that time, and spiced with a little obstacle-course flavor from new phenomena like the TV show *American Ninja Warrior*. It was a world away from the gym workouts we might have done ten years prior, where you'd work isolated body parts one at a time, loading weight onto stationary machines. This kind of garage-style workout fused rapid-fire drills that worked the whole body if you did it right — bodyweight moves like push-ups and pull-ups, explosive plyometric moves like box jumps and burpees, and strong-man moves swinging kettlebells and pushing weighted sleds. Cardio conditioning and strength-building were no longer separate entities; it all got covered at once. In contrast to chronic cardio training where you can easily zone out and spend a lot of time without getting a lot of effect, these circuit workouts were hard and fast, and once you got out the gate, they didn't let you dillydally around for a second.

The impact was immediate. When you combine strength plus speed you get a third quality: power. As our bodies got stronger, our endurance increased and so did our power to drive our bodies through space, even when loaded up with weight. This conditioned our cardiovascular systems and our metabolisms — the systems that turn food into energy — making them more efficient. A strength- and power-based workout can bring you to your knees by the end. What's wild is that even as you catch your breath and recover, splaying out in the awesome afterglow of tension that's releasing from every muscle fiber, your metabolism is continuing to work hard, burning calories stored as fat for up to forty-eight hours afterward. If you time your workouts wisely — not too many, not too few — and eat smartly alongside them (more on all that in chapters 6 and 7), the composition of your body begins to dramatically shift. Flabby fat stores get used up and, in their place, defined muscles appear. Under the surface, what's helping this happen is that the hormones regulating your blood sugar and storing and using calories are getting in shape, too, trained by the intense bursts of activity and rest. This means you are taking one of the best preventive health pills nature can dispense, improving insulin sensitivity and warding off chronic conditions like obesity and diabetes as well as turning around systemic inflammation (the precursor to many diseases), activating hormones that improve thinking and memory, and in my case, regulating blood pressure better. You are literally building a stronger state of health, from the inside out.

These "Gorilla Yard" workouts — so named because Dean thought our tires, ropes, and assorted objects for hurling and pounding looked like toys in a primate enclosure — became a ritual for us. We became converts to the ritual of physical exertion, loving the primal experience of digging deep past our comfort zones to discover grit on the other side, relishing moments to express raw feeling out loud, and embracing the high-frequency feeling we had when we hit the stage. None of us were drinking by this time, and though at first it was nerve-wracking to face the arena without the familiar haze, clearing the gunk, stress, and sluggishness out of our systems had a completely different effect. When you perform, you want to be a vessel for something bigger than yourself; call it inspiration, call it soul, or simply great music. By exerting yourself hard before a show, you propel energy and oxygen through every crevice, which clears out all the lines. Your vessel is cleaner and the message you're broadcasting — it can come out crystalline.

FROM STRENGTH TO POWER

Getting stronger and more powerful was game changing. I leaned out physically and leaned out in life. Making working out a priority required carving out time that nobody else could steal; this meant setting better boundaries around who and what got my attention. I started drawing stronger lines so that more of me went to the people who deserved it most — my wife and daughters. I like to think that as I carved away some of the deadweight physically, I did the same mentally. I literally had to slow the rush and edit the more, more, more ambition that drove me professionally in order to create space for my health. Gradually my family told me I was becoming better at listening, not just talking, and — with muscles tired out by midafternoon — better at simply sitting still and being present.

There's a funny thing about getting healthier. When you start experiencing what it's like to truly feel good, you want more of it. It can reach a point when you have to shake up your whole operating system. It can be a bumpy ride. Old ways of eating no longer sit right. Crutches and stimulants become jarring, not energizing — you want them out, too. It's like cotton wool is taken out of your ears; the muffle is gone and everything comes in clearer. Then you notice more of your surroundings as well: Is my environment supporting my goals or sabotaging them? Are the people I spend the most time with on board with this vision, or at odds with it? Luckily, Faith and the girls liked the benefits enough to accommodate my new routine with only a little grumbling and groaning about dad's workouts. The bigger issue was professional dissonance: While some members of my inner circle were stepping up the game to be as healthy and sharp as they could be, others were cruising on old check-out habits and enabling the party lifestyle to simmer on the sidelines. *Put your oxygen mask on first,* my wiser self told me, even though I tend to choose loyalty before logic sometimes. *Set up the conditions to be the best leader you can be.* What happened next caused some turbulence: I threw down the gauntlet to my band and my support team. "Guys, we're not getting any younger. The competition's not getting any easier. If we're gonna keep up, we need to step it up to be the best we can be — and I know in my heart that each one of you has it in you."

It didn't sit well with everyone. Gauntlet-throwing can be uncomfortable and not without pain. But the turnover that resulted let fresh growth burst forth. My band and I started bringing a whole new level of play to the table, more synced and cohesive than ever before. Our behind-the-scenes organization started hitting a flow as individuals got more in rhythm with each other. And that was the glue that held us together better. The fact that we all in some shape or form congregated at our makeshift church of fitness. Not everyone wanted to be a superathlete. Some dipped their toes into our workouts and took what they needed, or did their own thing entirely like yoga, but everyone shared a value: ownership of their physical and mental health.

Fitness can become a powerful team-building practice for a group, and it certainly did for the men and women I work with. We're all pretty competitive by nature.

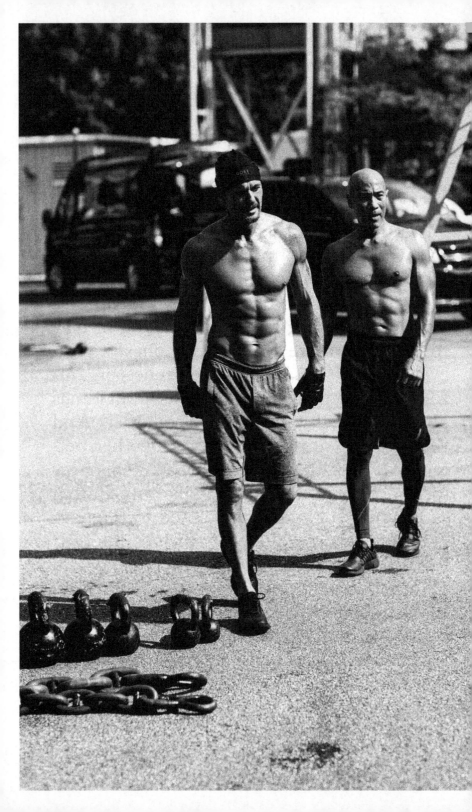

Giving that energy a chance to express itself physically changed our dynamic. When you've tensed and released your physical muscles, a mirror effect takes place within your mind: anxiety and frustrations subside, blame and judgment decrease, and time-wasting goes down. And getting sweaty together breaks down false barriers of ego or pride. When you've cheered someone through their thirtieth burpee or teamed up on a sled drag with them, you bring that same spirit of community and support to the meeting or studio. When it comes to Team McGraw, we have the added twist that nobody wants to be the weak link. We push each other to perform better, as music professionals but more important as people, and the healthful culture we built gels us as a team.

This turned out to be a good thing. About four years into this lifestyle the fight with my record label got uglier still and we found ourselves in court. Despite the stress this caused, I became even more focused on my goals. I was turning forty-five about then and the urgency hit me like a slap in the face: *You've got one shot at this gig. Your best concerts, music, movies — they're within reach. This is it. Go big or go home.*

My whole life, I've lived according to one

key value. I guess I've done so from an early age, when I wanted so fiercely to get beyond my circumstances. That value is, *Be ready.* Be primed for opportunity when it shows up, because it will come once, it will move on quick, and if you're not ready to make the shot, your whole destiny can change in a heartbeat. Miss that moment, and you'll live the rest of your life wondering just how much of your potential never played out.

That's when I decided to go from being in good shape to being in the best shape of my life.

ENTER THE DRAGON

In fitness, if you don't progress and evolve, you can plateau. Your body needs new stresses and challenges or it hits a point where progress stalls out; your body adapts to the demands you're putting on it, gets efficient at meeting them, and stops working so hard. You might be doing the same workout, but it's gotten easier for your body. Kind of like learning a language — after a while, it doesn't take as much effort to remember the vocabulary or conjugate the verbs. That means the health benefits of your workouts decrease a little unless you switch things up. You can also unknowingly overwork one aspect of your body without developing others, risking strain or injury. I didn't think I was plateauing until I met the man who turns men and women into superheroes.

How this occurred was kind of comical. I'd been watching the movie *Immortals,* in which Spartan warriors hurl themselves over battle gates and make mayhem with Greek weapons, their invincible torsos the epitome of manly strength. *These guys would kick that underwear model's butt,* I thought. I mused aloud, *What kind of genius trained these guys?* And my brilliant assistant took me seriously. Googling around and making some calls, she handed me a number — the perk of this line of business is that crazy things like this can actually happen. *This guy,* she said.

Enter Roger Yuan, one of my favorite true mavericks: former competitive martial artist; movie-fight coordinator and stunt man; part human, part panther. He's the man who prepares actors to flex, fight, and fall like ninjas and then shows the newbies how an O.G. does it, performing in movies like *Crouching Tiger, Hidden Dragon.* He's taught James Bond how to take down assassins looking flawless in a Tom Ford suit. Enough said.

Roger's older than I am but moves like he's ageless. Gravity has a different relationship with this guy; his center of power is so developed — in the Taoist wisdom tradition it's called the *dantien,* the area just below the navel — that he is a master of precise movement. His limbs whip out of nowhere or slice through space like a sword as his core rotates like a corkscrew, all parts moving as one unit with his feet light on the ground. It's total flow and awesome to watch. Both non-rule-book types, we have a lot in common — he feels like he's my brother from another mother — but Roger's a lot more philosophical than I am. Where my tendency is to go harder, go faster — always chased by those hungry ghosts telling me I haven't done enough work — Roger knows that power is sourced in stillness. The first time we worked out together, I put him through the killer three-part routine that I usually do solo before a big show, preparing like an athlete for a championship game. My ego got a buzz when Roger found a couch afterward and told everyone not to let me find him. But he soon had a comeback for me. Watching me move, he said, "Tim, you have white-boy hips."

Though I'd trained myself to be strong and fast, I was also as stiff as a board. I had the blocky strength of a sports player but was only enjoying a fraction of what my body could do. Roger dropped to the floor in a jiu jitsu move, balancing on one leg and one hand while sweeping the other leg low across the floor, popping back up in perfect control without a wobble. Then he dropped back down into a perfectly balanced pistol on the other foot, his full body weight supported on one deeply squatting leg, his butt almost touching the floor. "Wouldn't it feel great to be able to move like this onstage?" he asked. I tried to copy him and yelped. My hip flexors, calf muscles, and quads were too rigid to allow it, and the joints in my hips and ankle creaked and popped like rusty hinges. *Yes,* I managed to say.

Roger teaches that focusing on looks and musculature is a narrow view of fitness; the pliability of the muscles and the mobility of the joints are equally as important. In other words, flexibility and range of motion are as important as strength. So is being able to slow your roll enough to master movements well and breathe deeply and robustly, which seems innocuous but conditions your diaphragm and strengthens the core. We started transforming my body from stiff to supple, lengthening muscle tissues with yoga postures, restoring mobility to the joints, and nourishing connective tissues with animalistic moves that had me crawl, slither, and prowl across the floor. Stick fighting, boxing, and static horse stances taught me to find my center and work with gravity, developing agility and precision. Movements at odd angles and strange directions forced me to work neglected body parts and integrate them through a strong center. Roger loves to take an intensity addict like me and strip things back to basics. "Tai chi slow, Tim, tai chi slow," he'd say, directing me to master a safe and stable movement before allowing it to happen at speed. "We want you to still be doing this at ninety," he'd counsel, making me roll my spine and pelvis painfully over therapy balls to release the tensions that were compromising my technique. "As we get older, the tricks we used to meet high demands won't work; there's less margin for error." It was preventive medicine at work. And sometimes we'd change the stimuli to the body entirely by taking a workout to the pool, where water, not weights, became the element of resistance.

I'll confess right now that as good as this sounds, it didn't come easy to balance my fiery yang energy with Roger's Zen-like yin, where the goal is to be present in each moment and each movement, not just push through them. To this day my mind grapples with how eight good reps could be better than twenty (even though logically I know that eight reps done with perfect form and focused breath will put you right in the sweet spot). But the proof that I'd broken past the plateau was the way I functioned, felt, and looked. By doing this well-rounded style of functional fitness, I grew stronger and faster while entire ranges of motion that were unavailable to me before started to open up. I found myself dropping into a pistol mid-song onstage, having a moment with a fan in the front row, then pivoting back up easily, totally unaware of what I'd just done. I've always been a big mover onstage, but this opened it up to another level and I loved how fun it felt to have the confidence and comfort to truly let loose. Plus, who knows if anyone noticed, but my stronger diaphragm made me a better singer with a higher range as well.

And maybe most important of all, the improvements transferred to real life. Outside of workouts and performing, I discovered all the things I enjoyed doing most, like playing flag football with family and friends or spearfishing on vacation, got easier and better. By combining strength, power, newfound mobility and stability, and improved breathing, I could play harder, swim deeper, and not worry about throwing out a shoulder or knee. Putting these missing pieces into the mix felt like finally touching what

I'd longed for when I launched the fitness journey. I'd gotten control of my body, and that had allowed me to forget it — to feel free in any element, solid and light on my feet at once, trusting my body to carry me through.

Of course, I'd be remiss if I didn't acknowledge another nice benefit of developing well-rounded strength: getting dressed in the morning became easier than ever. There's probably not a man or woman alive who wouldn't agree that it feels pretty good to just throw on a pair of jeans and a T-shirt, confident that you don't need to "hide" anything underneath. It also doesn't suck when the fancier stuff — like that hand-tailored suit you've been eyeing — fits like a glove. What can I say? I'm a clothes horse. I think we're here on this earth to enjoy all of it — and getting in shape helped me enjoy it even more.

MIND, HEART, INSTINCT

It's been more than a decade since my dark night of the soul inspired my quest for health. Today our lifestyle in the McGraw household isn't exactly rock 'n' roll. Faith and I cook most of our food at home, and we're usually in bed by 9:30 p.m. — paying off those years of sleep debt — because a worked body is a tired body and my commitment to exercise every morning hasn't waned. If I'm at home, on tour, on a trip, or on vacation, I work out in some shape or form every day — sometimes playing a sport or some other recreational activity in addition. The way I work out on tour, when I want to build up to a certain persona before I get onstage, is intense. When I'm on vacation, on the other hand, I might tempt Faith or one of the girls to join me for some animal-flow moves and yoga sequences, topped with a few kettle-bell drills. (Though truth be told, I've been known to train for my vacations, too — like when I wanted to get in really good shape for a spearfishing and free-diving trip.) The general formula: Exercise daily, with some days more challenging than you'd like and other days gentler and restorative, or even quite passive to ensure you recover, then wrap that daily activity in a lifestyle of more movement.

The path to health can feel like one step forward and one step back at times. I'm no exception to the rule: I'll lose focus or moti-vation for a minute, or a week, or more. But now I recognize when that happens and have learned to expect both the A-plus days and the C-minus days, and chalk it up to being human. Life is peaks and valleys, and what matters is that you are self-aware enough to know your motivations, your quirks, and your weaker areas so that you can outwit yourself should your mind suddenly command you to ditch the trail. I'm still working on my weak spots, namely being kind to my body and believing that sometimes less can be more and rest can be best. But what's helped me stay the course is that I'm not a quitter. Getting healthy and fit is a bit like a marriage — you have to move beyond the initial infatuation, make a public commitment, and then show up to the relationship every day. You've got to have some friends helping you stay on track through the rough patches and trust that even when it's hard, the sum total of your efforts will endure and sustain you like almost nothing else.

Recently I looked up the definition of the word *integrity*. It has three meanings: the state of being whole; being of sound, unimpaired condition; and having ethics and moral character. I like to think that my decade of physical practice has been a journey of integrating my body so it functions efficiently and effectively as a strong and dynamic whole. It's also been a journey from a man who was a little bit rocky — fractured and slightly broken — to a person, father, and husband of more integrity, one who's still working on it and still fumbling it from time to time. I can't say I've "arrived" anywhere, because the humbling truth is you are always on the journey and life will inevitably show up to highlight what you haven't yet mastered. But my physical practice has helped me "work out" some of what stood in my way.

I like the way that Roger states his philosophy on fitness. He's said, *To be able to move well is to be physically fit; to be able to move and breathe well under stress is to be emotionally and physically fit; to be able to move well, think, and have maximal perception as well as problem-solving ability, as well as the capacity to be emotionally both empathetic and emotionally secure — that's the combination of all three: strength of mind, strength of heart, strength of instinct. All of those things can't happen if your body is weak.*

I don't know if I'd have had the insight to say it like that, but I wholeheartedly agree with Roger. So much of what's right in life starts with a strong, healthy body.

You might read all this and think, *It's great that this routine works for you, but I'm not athletic, and it wouldn't work for me.* I urge you to reconsider. *Athlete* just means someone with a physical practice — and that can take on many different forms. I started by simply

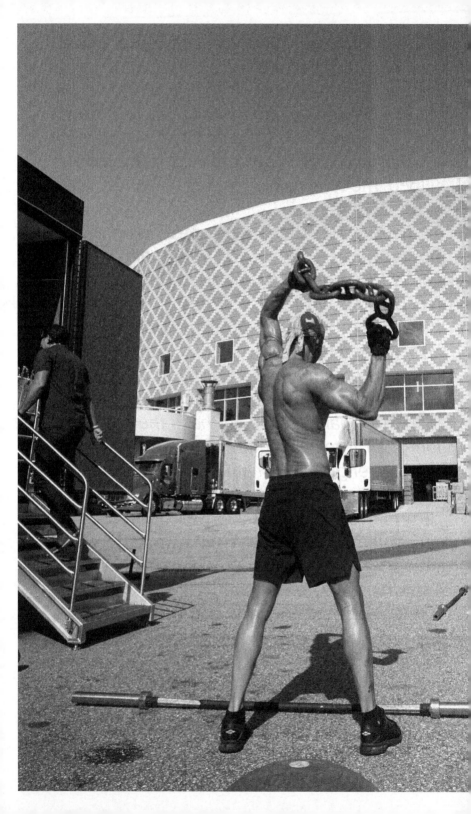

committing to getting that first foot on the floor. I graduated to having both feet firmly on the floor. And now I stand more centered in life, less buffeted by the storms and dramas, and more tuned in on a daily basis to the state of my mind, heart, and instinct. The funny thing about it all? It began with a pair of tennis shoes, a daily walk, and — as I like to joke — a good old attitude of high hopes and low expectations.

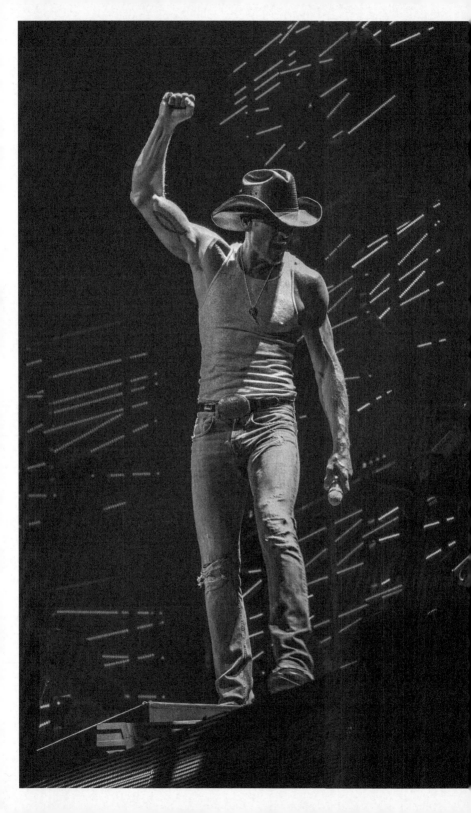

CHAPTER 2

A MAVERICK'S MANIFESTO

Now's the moment I get to hop up onto my soap box. You know why staying fit is important to me. But why should it matter to you? Give me a few minutes and let me be your training instigator, your healthy habit cheerleader — the person who lights the fire in you to make daily movement central to your life. It's not my style to sermonize, but when you land on something that has such potential to turn your life around, it'll make you want to preach a little.

I believe that, as individuals and as a society, we're at a moment of reckoning. We've watched as the pace of life has accelerated exponentially and stress levels have gone through the roof. Technology has staged a takeover of our minds while our bodies have become unnaturally sedentary. We're being forced to go hard in the parts of life — working nine to five, or six, or seven — that don't necessarily bring the most fulfillment.

Add to this the fact that families today live farther apart than ever before, and traditional support groups don't exist in the way they did a few generations ago, and it becomes easy to see why so many people feel overwhelmed and disconnected. And then there's the nonstop onslaught of information, comparison, and round-the-clock news. If you're feeling sick, tired, and stressed out, you're not on the fringes — you're in the majority.

Call it burnout culture, call it convenience culture, call it on-demand culture; it's turned all of our regular rhythms and the values we once held dear on their heads. We work extra-long days and sit for hours in transit before and after. Fast food is often more affordable and accessible than real food. Nature's least expensive medicine, eight hours' sleep, is a luxury. Moving our bodies in a way that makes us stronger has somehow become expensive and complicated. And the most "connected" generation ever is also being called the loneliest generation ever. Little by little, the pillars that hold up our physical health have started to buckle. And the consequences aren't limited to our bodies. They move upward — badly straining our mental and emotional states. Because our bodies and our minds are not isolated entities, they are two parts of one whole, each affecting the other.

Here's the good news: I think this crisis point is also a pivot point. We're waking up to the price of our super-modern lifestyle and getting motivated about finding our own way through it, refusing to let it exact such a toll. Why do I think this? Well, being a recording artist gives you some interesting insight into the human condition. I make songs about very human things — the way we live and the way we love, our most private hopes and our most public regrets. Maybe because I sing from the heart, I get heartfelt feedback in response. What I'm sensing is a wave of change rolling in to shore. Times are turbulent and we might disagree about a lot of things, but it sure feels like we're coming to consensus that it's time to reclaim owner-ship of our lives, starting with our physical and mental health, our relationships to oth-ers, and our deeper connection to purpose, meaning, and truth. We've stretched the elastic band to its limit, and now we have a choice: pull it till it breaks, or let it go a little and find some slack. And nobody benefits when your physical or mental health snaps.

That doesn't mean that change is easy — actually, it's the opposite. Change can be unsettling, partly because it requires effort and partly because it's so comfortable to disengage and move through life on autopilot, to order in instead of cooking from scratch, to duck out of sight in real life but show up on social media, all filtered and flawless. Yet doing more of the same isn't working, and it's not making us happy or healthy. We've come a long way from what our grandparents and great-grandparents understood: Real satisfaction in life comes from doing the effortful thing. Working hard, cooking (even growing) real food, getting through the grind with support from others, standing up for what's right and taking care of what needs to be done even when you don't particularly want to do it. And look at photos of those folks — everyday Americans in the 1940s, '50s, '60s (or even later depending on your age). Tell me, do they not, on average, look leaner, healthier, happier, and less puffy than we do?

If you picked up this book, chances are you want to make a change. Maybe you feel stuck in a cycle of dissatisfaction like I was or even numbed out or apathetic. It's easy to beat yourself up about feeling this way, and it's so important to know that part of your emotional response is based on biology. One thing I've learned in the process of getting healthier is that when your brain produces less dopamine (aka, the feel-good "reward" chemical), which is released when you do something enriching and meaningful, you're not going to feel awesome. Dopamine imbalance happens when you haven't been active — and especially if your recreation involves sedentary and ultra-stimulating stuff like gaming and social media. Don't worry: Establishing positive habits will turn around that imbalance, and an exercise ritual will help springboard you out of apathy.

Maybe you are frustrated or even angry that situations in your life make it challenging to have the time and resources to take care of yourself in the way you need and deserve. I say, *feel* that. Let that frustration serve as the fuel to your fire that ignites positive changes. In some shape or form we all hit those walls, and it's easier to burst through them when you don't fight the feelings, but use them to your advantage to propel you off the couch to blaze your own trail and hold a torch up high. What helps is knowing that if you feel this way, you're far from alone.

Whenever I hit a problem, I'm not quite sure how to deal with, like helping my kids when they're having a tough time or getting relationships on track when they've gone a bit awry, I look for the best advice I can find. I'll read snippets from all kinds of experts, mining their work for nuggets that can help me show up better. And you know the theme I've seen repeated most often, from all kinds of angles and very different voices? It's pretty consistent. When you're in trying times or caught in a tailspin, do two things first: Change your state physically, and connect with others. Moving more, not thinking more, is the way in to making things better. Reaching out, not retreating, is the path to a happier state.

Right around the time I sat down to write this chapter, I had an experience I never would have envisioned back when I was a kid in Start, Louisiana, riding my bike past the bayou and doing backflips with my buddies into cotton trucks. I got to work out with my best friends and bandmates at the launch of a training studio I helped to create near my home in Nashville. The facility is called TRUMAV Fitness. The "mav" conjures up the word *maverick,* and the studio is stocked with all the crazy stuff we've put together for full-body, functional-fitness-style training, scaled to be accessible for everyone: the beginner and the advanced athlete alike, the high schooler and the retiree. But it wasn't the ropes, weight bags, and balance balls that struck me as we walked in to get our butts whooped (while cameras rolled, filming it for posterity). It was the paragraph that had been stenciled on the wall in the entrance hall to catch your eye the minute you walk in. It's kind of fitness call to arms. Here's how it reads:

A TRUMAV shows up every day, focuses on the goal, defies the odds, encourages others, puts in the time, works hard, then works harder, overcomes obstacles, envisions the future, embraces the grind, believes everyone is worthy of a healthy life, dreams big, answers to something greater, remains resilient despite challenges, shows courage in the face of adversity, works hard for results, trusts we are stronger together, gives their all.

The rallying call got me feeling as pumped

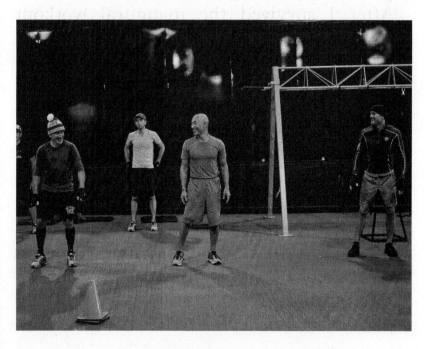

as Rocky running up his Philadelphia steps. It was January and just like anyone else whose family goes big on holiday food, I needed the jump-start to turn the corner and get back into tour shape. But you know what hit me the most as I looked at those words? The fact that none of them touched on the idea of having a perfect body or being an all-star athlete. In fact, they weren't about the external rewards or prizes at all. They made the case that the true reason to commit to a fitness practice is to hone yourself from the inside out: to build a strong mind and feel braver in the face of challenge, to find out what you're made of and inspire you to live bigger than you might otherwise.

After I survived the inaugural workout with a studio full of women and men of all ages, experience levels, and body types, sweating together through the intervals and making it intact to the other side, I felt the energy of the room skyrocket. And it hit me even harder: The fundamental reason we all show up to train our bodies is really very simple. We can use it as a tool to blast past inner obstacles and shut up the voices that tell us, "You can't do that." We can use it as a tool to feel a connection with other people, to feel grounded in a community. Whether a person ever achieves Iron Man or Woman status or gets as sleek as a human racehorse is almost beside the point. That stuff, should it happen, is the happy aftereffect of tending to your body and mind.

Roger likes to remind us, as we tremble our way through a tough exercise or try to rush past the warmup to get to the fun stuff of throwing things at each other, "Breathe and stay with it; the body will come; the 'runner's high' will come, but don't chase the outer prizes. Just practice being present to your self. In an age of distraction, temptation, and increasing anxiety, the idea of using fitness to come back to yourself is even more important than ever. Moving your body primes you to do better and give more in every area of your life. I want you to jump on my bandwagon — whether you've never seen yourself as athletic or whether you could out-burpee me before breakfast. So listen up." Here, in the most simplified version possible, is my down-and-dirty five-point manifesto for why moving daily matters so much.

#1: YOU START AN UPWARD SPIRAL
When I took the bull by the horns and started my big dig into a fitter lifestyle, the first side effect from hitting the gym consistently was this: My cravings for unhealthy

food switched to cravings for healthy food. As I got my energy back and felt my body kick into higher gear again, I wanted to fill it with everything the old me had nimbly avoided. Suddenly, I was craving big green salads instead of avoiding them, and grabbing handfuls of almonds as snack instead of handfuls of candy. I looked forward to a nice piece of fish seared on the grill and served with my favorite vegetables. And this coming from a guy who has eaten his fair share of late-night takeout.

Not only that, but I finally became friends with water in a way I'd never anticipated. Water! The element we most take for granted — the liquid that coffee and beer drinkers mainly acknowledge as the basis of their brew. This part of the health equation took me a minute. How can something as simple as drinking water all day be difficult? Dumb as it sounds, it's always been a problem for me. It took me a few hard lessons in dehydration, including one very public collapse onstage in Europe, to fully understand how lots of caffeine, hours of air travel, plus intense workouts could add up to do a number on the hydration of the body. After that, I changed course. I started consuming a lot more water, and it worked wonders. When your hydration is optimized, the turnaround can be a 180. Drinking enough water boosts energy and brainpower, helps to balance out your blood pressure, flushes out toxins and get things moving in your gut, keeps you feeling full and satiated, and hydrates your skin (aka, fewer wrinkles). More water delivers all those things and more.

As for the part of the health equation that a lot of experts now say is *the* most important part of your lifestyle to change — maybe even more important than exercise and diet — I began to sleep more, dragged into slumber by a squad of tired muscles. And when I slept better, I woke up more refreshed and in a better frame of mind, as Faith would probably attest. My rested brain made better choices the next day, felt less tempted by roller-coaster foods and drinks — like super-strong coffee to get things going that'll make you crash a few hours later.

The more I stayed on the path, the more smoothly a positive feedback loop moved through every area of my life. When you eat a diet full of fresh vegetables and free of processed foods and cheap restaurant cooking oils, your gut health is improved and your digestion works better, sending more nutrition into your cells. In conjunction with all the water, sleep, and vigorous movement, eating plenty of vegetables helps keeps everything moving along smoothly. The better your cells uptake the good stuff from food, the more energy you have and the better foods' vitamins and minerals get absorbed to strengthen your immune system. You don't get sick as often, and you have more energy to work out. And if you can clear out foods that have an inflammatory effect on the body, like sugar, excess pasteurized dairy, and — if you're sensitive to them — grains, you might suddenly notice, as I did, that soreness and stiffness go down a hundredfold as a result. With fewer aches and pains, you're even more inspired to continue on your healthier path. And did I mention being just a little less cranky? Well, that's what they tell me.

You probably get the drift. It's as if, without you necessarily *trying* to overhaul your lifestyle, and without obsessing about it and driving yourself to distraction about it, a clean-up crew quietly does some work, taking some of the worst stuff out and slipping better stuff in its place. You trade bad addictions for better addictions — the kind that may require a little time and knife skills to prepare but make you feel a whole lot better. And all this output from a single input: exercising daily. Putting one foot in front of the other — literally, it can be that simple — or

Stress and caffeine have a codependent relationship. Get tired and depleted from stress, sleep poorly, and there's a pretty good chance you'll crave caffeine within minutes of waking up. Listen, a great cup of coffee is no bad thing in my opinion — it can be part of a deeply satisfying ritual that not only helps you feel more alert but also gives you the chance to pause for a few minutes and focus on your goals for the day. Plus, the bitter compounds in coffee beans are actually health-promoting. The problem is when we use strong caffeine as a crutch. (And when servings get supersized — have you ever seen how small a coffee cup was in the 1950s?) Our bodies respond to caffeine with an adrenaline surge. Adrenaline is a hormone that is released in the body when we perceive danger — it and its sister hormone, cortisol, mobilize us to survive by any means necessary by making emergency energy available to our muscles. If you're already worn down, any kind of stress becomes incredibly taxing on the body, exhausting its reserves. That's when throwing caffeine into your system too often can add to the burden, causing fatigue that you feel deep in your bones and can't be easily shaken. (Not to mention some people metabolize caffeine quickly, whereas in other people it sticks around longer, disrupting sleep even more that night.) If you love coffee or strong black tea, beware of the false energy it offers and try making one (moderate-sized) cup really count. Have it early before mid-morning and savor it; then if you're craving more, switch to a coffee alternative — there are lots of herb and super-herb blends out there today. And if you slump midafternoon, good news, you have a healthier alternative than making a run to the espresso hut: stand up, jump, run, or lift. Even a couple minutes of exercise will boost your energy in a much more sustainable way. If you're still tired after that, for God's sake take a nap or plan for an early bedtime. Your body's crying for rest.

as your ability grows, getting your chin above a bar and your butt down to your heels.

In health circles they would probably say that what I did was lay down a *keystone habit*. A keystone is the stone that sits at the summit of an arch, locking the whole structure in place. Likewise, a keystone habit is one good habit you lay down in your life around which other good habits start to orbit. If you can get that center stone in place, it makes getting in the groove with other good ones happen a lot more naturally.

I've seen similar things occur many times over as friends and bandmates fall into our fitness vortex. They start working out, get the bug for it, and next thing you know they're bringing salad in a jar to the rehearsal studio when everyone else is chewing on burritos and drinking Coke. In extreme cases — like our guitarist Denny — they become a paragon of health, with grass-fed butchers on speed dial and a thriving side business as a nutritional coach.

Here's why I think daily exercise is more powerful than any other intervention you could start with on the path to better health — more than pledging to go on a diet, even. It's one small thing that you can do immediately, without overhauling your pantry, mastering recipes, or fighting off the urge to buy chips. It might only start with a morning or evening walk. But what happens *during* that walk is much bigger than it seems. Moving your body starts to reverse the energy deficit and low morale that might have crept in from another long day of sitting down and putting out fires or holding down the fort. Everyone knows the physical collapse that happens when you haven't been active; your posture goes concave and your spine rolls forward, your neck juts out as you stare at a screen and your chair-bound hips start to feel like concrete. Your breath gets shallow, as if you are barely breathing at all. It's a picture of restriction: You actually seem to shrink a little, as everything slumps inward and down. A plethora of research shows that this kind of body posture creates a mind-set of defeat; you feel robbed of power. When your head is tipping downward, it's a lot harder to see what's possible. Remember back in physics class they taught Newton's first law of motion? It goes like this: A body at rest will remain at rest unless an outside force acts on it. Forget to get up, and no wonder apathy sets in.

But don't call the undertakers just yet. The flip side of this situation is that getting up and moving can turn the slow landslide around.

Standing up tall and getting moving automatically starts to reverse the low mojo moment. Swinging your arms and legs as you walk presses restart on your nervous system, and breathing deeper to power the movement pumps more oxygen into your tissues and wakes up the sluggish brain. You start to think a little more clearly. As sticky joints start to move in their sockets, lubricating fluids get flushed around them, and you begin to loosen up. Movement boosts circulation, which means that everything required for health goes where it needs to go — the nutrients and hormones carried in the blood get to the tissues and organs that need them, and the waste materials held in the lymph — the fluid that clears out toxins — get processed and released. The cumulative effect: It feels better to be in your body, which makes it feel better to be in your mind . . . which makes it feel a hell of a lot better to be you. The more energized body is now driving the mind *up*. Movement of any kind, even low-impact stuff like walking, will boost serotonin and endorphins, the feelgood chemicals that improve your mood. It also improves your brain's ability to make new connections — to make sense of the world differently. And though you can't see it happen, under the surface you're creating conditions for the body to take back control.

The effects of this upward spiral get even better if you exercise outside, because not only does daylight hitting your skin and eyes help to counteract the health-crushing

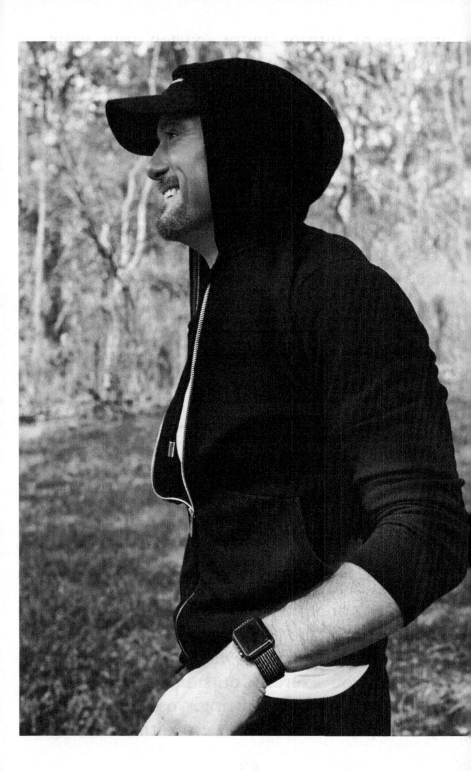

impact of being inside in front of a screen, you also get a boost of well-being from nature. It can feel isolating and demoralizing when you're inactive or worse, when you feel stuck in a body you're convinced doesn't love you. The act of moving your body outside even in the smallest, least Instagramable way makes you feel less isolated in the world, whether your companions are trees, birds, passersby, or playful dogs running laps around you. Take it up a notch and get walking or exercising with others and you really get on a roll, boosting your health further from a sense of connection and camaraderie. Plus, exercising with others helps to reinforce your healthy lifestyle so that it's less of a stretch; it starts to feel like the thing everybody does, so why wouldn't you? And as you continue on the spiral up, your brain secretes more and more dopamine — in advance of doing the exercise, or eating the healthy meal, or slipping into your sleep routine. With time, if this happens enough, the good-for-you habits become more persuasive than the bad-for-you habits, and the upward spiral continues. Your arch gets even stronger as the keystone and all the supporting stones around it lock firmly into place.

It's funny how often people ask me, "How do you do your workouts and still have energy for the show?" I tell them it's *because* of the workouts that we feel so exuberant. Our workouts get our systems revving at a higher level, buzzing with energy, which bounces off the stage and out there to the audience. The burn we built in the afternoon sustains to the show. So get out there, even if you're not ready to get after it yet. A life-changing year can start with a simple walk around the block.

#2: YOU PURGE STRESS AND COMBAT ANXIETY

Have you ever gotten so into singing along to a song, you purge pent-up emotions and release all the stuff that's been weighing you down? Playing music has always done that for me; it's cathartic to build up momentum as I sing. There's so much intensity in the playing that any negative emotions get churned around like a washing machine, then ricochet out of my body and into the night sky. It leaves me feeling lighter — purified somehow. I'm pretty sure that if I do my part right, you get to experience it, too. It's what bonds us together at a show — we let the music move us.

Working out is cathartic in a similar way. Movement helps all kinds of toxins circulate more freely so they can get processed and released. To my mind this includes mental and emotional toxins just as much as physical ones.

Even though stress seems like a mental phenomenon that takes over your mind with a vise grip, it's a deeply physical phenomenon. When the brain perceives a situation as threatening or too hard to handle, it sets off the release of a series of hormones that prompt the secretion of adrenaline and cortisol, our primary stress hormones. Though adrenaline disperses rapidly, cortisol likes to hang around in the bloodstream for longer, especially if you sit all day and don't help move it out — literally. Movement, along with enough sleep, is a good way to keep elevated cortisol levels in check. When cortisol lingers, it starts making a mess of things: it can raise blood pressure and blood sugar, lead to weight gain (especially in your midsection), make it hard to think straight and even harder to sleep, impair your body's ability to repair from illness or injury, and make you hyperreactive to stressful demands — even small stressors start to trigger an outsize physiological stress response, exhausting your reserves further. This cycle, not surprisingly, starts to color the way you see the world and can contribute to depression. And when you're tired, stressed, angry, and gaining weight, it's all too easy to self-medicate to help take the edge off with sugar, alcohol, or other kinds of crutches. Most of which — no surprise here — elevate cortisol higher.

Not only does it feel bad mentally to be stressed out, but being stressed out makes your body feel horrible: negative or painful situations cause you to tighten up your muscles and seal tension right into your tissues. If you've ever had someone knead stress out of your shoulders like a master baker pounding dough, you know how that goes. This can be a nuisance or it can be as disruptive as any other kind of injury, pulling your spine into misalignment, giving you back pain, pinching nerves, and a whole lot more. It's human nature to want to lock hard feelings out of sight, but stored tension can build up to the point where it can make you sick if you let it. Especially today, when any of us can feel a month's worth of stress just making it through a Monday.

My approach: Keep clearing out the closets on a regular basis so they don't explode open and dump their contents on you and the unsuspecting folks around you.

There are many ways to do this. Meditation is a good one for a lot of people. I'll have to work on that, though, because sitting still isn't my normal M.O. Working out is my way of working things out. Especially in the functional fitness style I've adopted. Lifting, throwing, and pulling stuff will get you back into your body in a primal way quick if your head's spinning out. If you give your body a chance to unlock the frozen-stuck parts and turn up your inner temperature, you'll find that once you warm up your tissues, they won't let you keep stress stuffed away. Working out with a group of people all grunting and groaning does wonders: It's like going up to the top of a mountain to wail and cry. You exorcise some of those negative energies by physically shaking them off, watching them lose steam as they move through and out. And if there are some hard feelings you've been avoiding, get ready. Heating up your body can bring them to a boil. But it's healthy: they can evaporate and condense, and then you leave them on the floor in a puddle of sweat.

Meanwhile, and so importantly, exercising helps your body create a cocktail of positive chemistry that lifts your mood, suppresses pain, and alleviates depression — chief among them, endorphins that give you the euphoric "runner's high" as well as mood-regulating serotonin, motivation-lifting dopamine, and alertness-boosting

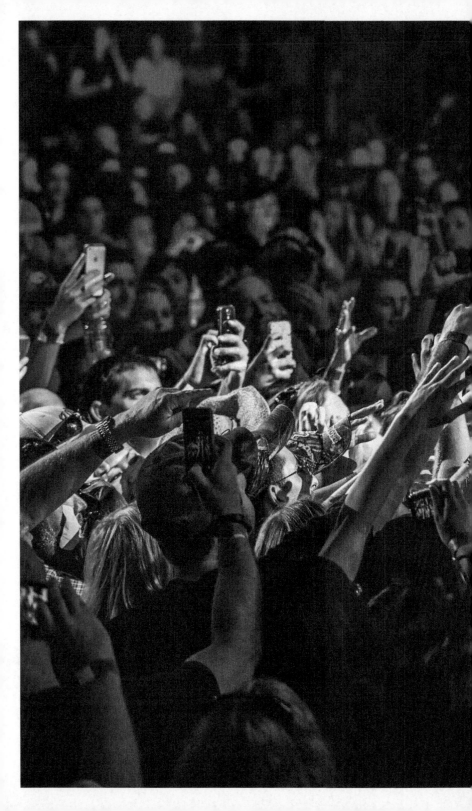

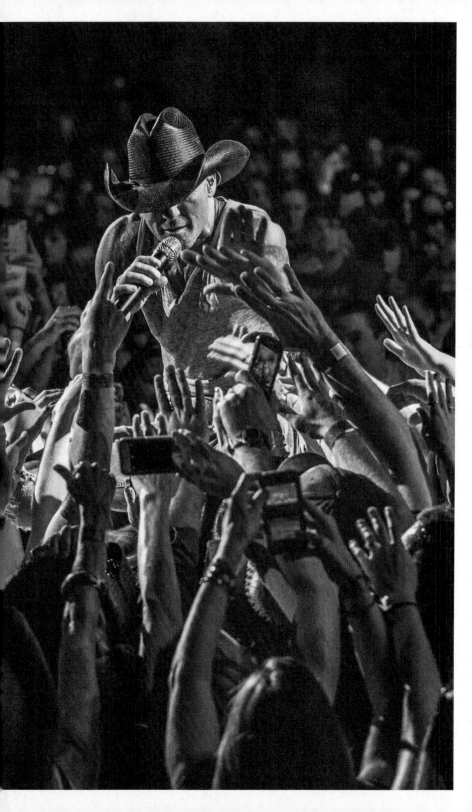

It can be tough to drag your body out of bed for an early morning walk or run, but if you've ever done it you know — once you're out the door and moving, you feel incredible. There's a reason for that: being outdoors has a therapeutic effect on our stressed-out minds and bodies, and exposure to the early morning sun is particularly beneficial. When we spend too much time indoors under artificial lights, our bodies' natural rhythms — which are set to the light-dark cycle of a twenty-four-hour day — become out of sync.

This gets especially turned around when we stay in our brightly lit homes as the world outside falls dark. Light from almost all indoor lighting plus the screens of devices is predominantly made up of frequencies of blue light, which nature only gives us when the sun is high in the sky in the middle of the day. When we're exposed to it before sunrise and after sunset, that kind of blue light scrambles all the signaling in our bodies, disrupting the way hormones work and energy gets made. At those times, our bodies would rather be bathed in the red frequencies of a rising or setting sun, of campfires and candles — or no light at all — than fake blue light. Taking care to reduce blue light exposure after dark is one powerful way to offset this (see page 394) and so is getting outside early to let early-dawn red light work its magic. As the study of "circadian biology" is now revealing, the first light of day literally helps to keep your biological clock on track, which affects everything from the quality of your sleep to your weight to your ability to grow new muscle. This clock also helps set your mood-boosting, health-repairing hormones to the levels required to stay well. So get out for your walk before sunrise, and if you're fortunate to live somewhere that the sun breaks over the horizon, let its light gently wash over your face (no sunglasses — you want the light to indirectly fill the receptors in your eyes).

norepinephrine. Of course, the mere fact of being around other people, all gathered around a positive, life-affirming common cause, is stress-relieving in itself. It's a loneliness antidote.

I don't want to imply that exercise is a

magic bullet or something that solves all your problems. You still have to solve your problems. But if you deploy the release valve regularly, it's one thing to help stay a step ahead of your shadows. It puts you in a better spot to handle things the way you know you *should* handle them, but sometimes spectacularly fail to do when the wolves of stress are hounding you and banging down the door. My daughters will hopefully attest to this — I got significantly better at being present for them in the way they needed once I was clearing my own stress through exercise, day in and day out. Plus, it turns out that when you flush out stress hormones, you bring a lot of other hormones back into balance, improving your total health. Your hormonal system is like an intricate, interconnected web. An imbalance in one place, like your stress response, can create an imbalance in another — like metabolism — at the drop of a hat. Correct the stress, and you can correct a lot more than your temperament.

It's amazing how many things in life go better when you don't fly off the handle at the slightest trigger. I've had a chance to test out this thesis roughly 3,650 times in the last decade and I know this to be true: I'm a much happier and more even-tempered person if I've had a great workout in the morning.

#3: YOU DEVELOP GRIT AND FORGE FOCUS

Picture this: it's an overcast fall afternoon in Cleveland, Ohio, and our touring caravan rolled in and set up camp for a stop on Faith's and my worldwide Soul2Soul tour. My hardy crew of fitness enthusiasts and I throw on our hoodies and eye the sky — dark clouds are brewing and the conditions don't look amenable for our daily workout on the blacktop. Shortly after our warm-up and midway into our first round of conditioning, rain starts to bucket down, drenching our clothes, shoes, and gear. The battle ropes we undulate to get our hearts racing and whip our upper bodies into shape instantly double in weight, saturated with water. Rivers run down our necks, soaking our skin. And instead of running for cover, we grimace a little, laugh a little, and dig in deeper. It's only a few minutes of our lives, after all.

Second snapshot of what some would call insanity: Albuquerque, New Mexico, on a sweltering summer afternoon. The expected midday monsoon hasn't hit, and the heat has broken triple digits. Foolishly, I grab the metal bar we use for a nasty sequence of overhead presses I call the Bar Complex — it's so hot I get blisters on my palms. (I never did that again.) Misstep rectified with a pair of powerlifting gloves, we get to it: a curtailed workout done with extra attention on staying hydrated, but a daily session nonetheless. (Truth be told, I then tried to get the guys to play pickup basketball after, but they wisely declined.)

Looking back at those two scenes of deluge and drought, what was going on was more than physical conditioning. We could have skipped those days and performed reasonably well onstage nonetheless. But we did them because they gave us a training ground for a set of skills that everyday life doesn't always give you chance to practice: to get uncomfortable, stop thinking, start doing, and build some grit.

Grit to me is a combination of focus and perseverance. You call on grit to keep yourself gunning for a personal cause that really matters to you when your ego is telling you to give up or downgrade your ambitions. Ditto for when naysayers doubt your capacities. Grit is what you tap into when you step up and stay in the game because it's the right thing to do, even when every cell in your body is yelling in resistance that it's not the

One reason that moving your body helps reverse anxiety and stress is that it forces you to breathe deeply. When you're sedentary, distracted, and stuck in your head, it's easy to fall into patterns of tight, constricted breathing or taking shallow gulps of air, both of which signal to your body a "fight or flight" stress response and prevent your parasympathetic nervous system — the part of your nervous system responsible for the smooth, regulated functioning of all your organs and systems — from running the way it should. You also deprive your tissues of oxygen. Roger's had to teach me the value of breath work because, like a lot of people, I feel too busy to give it its due. He literally had to tell me to stop holding my breath! But now we start workouts with a few minutes of "active breathing." You can use this tool anytime to invigorate your body, combat stress and anxiety, and "warm up" your tissues before working out by getting circulation going.

Roger's Breathing Exercise

Lie down comfortably on the floor with your arms by your sides, palms up or down, belly relaxed, tongue gently against roof of mouth. Breathe in slowly through nose to the count of five, allowing your rib cage to expand out and up and your belly to softly rise and fall. Visualize your diaphragm being pushed down by the volume of air entering your lungs. If you hear a few small cricks and cracks, that's good, it's just your body telling you that you're making more space. Pause at the fullest point of the breath for a count of two, then slowly exhale out of the nose, envisioning the diaphragm return to its relaxed "dome" shape as the air leaves your lungs. Repeat for at least one minute and up to five minutes. If you want, invite your body to release any tension and anxiety with each exhale and allow peace and space to enter with each inhale.

fun thing to do. Grit is what you draw from to do three things I value so deeply I have them scrawled on my gym mirror and underlined in black: *Never Give Up. Never Give Up. Never Give Up.*

I don't mean to sound extremist, or create the impression that this a lifestyle only for adrenaline junkies. Let's put it in a more relatable way. Developing a little grit helps you get a grip. When anyone asks to what I attribute success, I always say *focus* — the practice of putting my attention on the immediate task at hand and giving it 100 percent. Anytime things haven't gone well, professionally or personally, or when I haven't felt good about myself, has been when I've lost focus on what I wanted to accomplish. Focus is a mental skill, but you practice it with physical actions and choices — you decide every day where you want to invest your energy. It's like making your bed first thing in the morning. Faith schooled me in the habit. She said, "Just do your side, it won't take long." And now I feel like a kid getting a gold star each time I do it. It's not exactly gritty, but it's a good metaphor for working out. With one small physical action I'm training my brain to direct my attention where I want it, pressing pause on what I'd prefer to do to meet a higher goal of order. And I'm convinced that my one-minute tussle with my comforter sets the day off in a positive direction.

The irony is that today we give away our attention like it's worthless. We so easily fall into an internet rabbit hole or scroll endlessly on social media, hopping from one bright flashing screen to another like toy poodles jumping on command. We've forgotten the first law of success: Put your attention where you want it to go.

These days I'm updating my answer about success. Just about anything good that's happened in my life has come on the back of a second skill that's taken equal cultivation: perseverance. Where focus locks you into a task in the first place, perseverance keeps you working on the task through thick and thin, helping you see it through to completion. Without perseverance, circumstances will easily get the better of you. When something happens to test your mettle you can wilt a little and feel unable to step up to bat. In my case, that something was years of exhausting and stressful legal wrangling that kept testing my energy and resolve — it almost felt like something was drawing my life blood from my body. And if I hadn't trained for it, it might very well have gotten the better of me.

I am not a natural when it comes to these skills — I've put in the work to cultivate them so that I'm able to sustain my sanity, my integrity, and my health when tough situations arise. And though I know there are gentler ways to get there, the way I do it is cruder: training mental muscles alongside the physical ones, putting both sets to the test on the asphalt or the stadium stairs to find out what I'm made of. In other words, getting gritty.

One of my workout buddies told me about an article he'd read that said regular exercise is as effective as meditation in helping you build self-control and willpower. I have to say, I've seen these qualities skyrocket for me, and I believe it's because a workout habit done right really does hone your focus. Sticking with a routine and practicing that routine over and over, day in and day out, greases the groove in your brain that's in charge of drowning out distraction and grinding out the effort so you get the job done. Especially when you push your own boundaries and do things that are harder than you'd like. Pick up something heavy, hold a pose for longer than you think you can, do four circuits of a workout instead of three. Grappling a heavy sandbag or trembling in tai chi stance is a crude method of bringing your attention to the now — even if your mind is screaming, "I wanna stop!" It is fully present nonetheless, and there's not a millimeter of mental bandwidth left to think about tomorrow's to-do list. Even if you don't realize it, in those physically demanding situations you're retraining your brain to lock in to what's happening in the present moment instead of fixating on the past or worrying about the future. It supercharges the part of you that notices the now because every sensation gets amplified. If you can let go of wanting to be somewhere else and be *with* the feeling, working out can be its own form of sweaty meditation.

I live by the motto *Tough times don't matter; tough people do.* It means we can't always change our circumstances, but we can make ourselves more resilient and able to deal with challenges. And for me that starts with building a sound body and, in so doing, building a sound mind. What's interesting is that the benefits are the product of an interesting quirk in our human design: the body and brain grow in capacity when they experience positive stress; in other words, we *need* challenge to help us get to the next level, where we can handle *more* complexity and demands.

So make the backyard or living room your dojo. Stop giving in to instant gratification for a minute. Don't look for "likes" or cruise other peoples' feeds. Flex and hone the mental muscles of focus and perseverance while you make your physical muscles burn. That stronger mind-set will be there for you in the good times, helping you stick with a healthy lifestyle. And, maybe more important, in the bad times, too.

#4: YOU CREATE CONFIDENCE THROUGH ACTION

Let me tell you the story of Billy Nobel, our charming and talented keyboardist. The first day Billy came on tour with the band as a slender young guy of twenty-nine years, he wasn't in bad shape, but — and I say this with love — he was like a lot of musicians, great at their craft but physically reminiscent of the guy in the Charles Atlas cartoon getting sand kicked in his face. Billy saw our workout crew getting suited up for a run, talking smack to each other as we warmed up, and he turned pale. He thought, *I'm doomed! McGraw won't keep me around because I don't work out!* That would never have happened, because Billy's an incredible guy with a real musical gift. But I do remember thinking he was ripe for a makeover.

That first day, Billy stood a little forlorn at the loading dock when we returned from the run, handing out water so we'd know he cared about our mission. His hesitancy didn't last long. At Team McGraw we pride ourselves on equal opportunity workouts; the daily sessions on the blacktop are open to any member of the tour family who has the time and inclination to participate, and the original members mentor any new recruits so they ramp up safely without overstraining themselves. Billy decided that we old guys — at least one of us thirty years older than he — might just know something he didn't, so he joined in.

At first, Billy could barely flip a tire and he couldn't do a single pull-up. But motivated by the group, he kept showing up and gradually gained strength and endurance. A few weeks into his new habit, Billy had a shock when he looked in the mirror: His love handles were gone and in their place were visible obliques. That minor moment triggered a significant inner shift. Billy said that all his life he'd felt uneasy in his body — he was on the enviably skinny side but was undefined and soft, and he'd never actually liked what he saw. Seeing the love handles fade out as his trunk, glutes, and hips started cranking, and then seeing his arms take shape was a powerful wake-up. He discovered, *I don't have to accept what I'm not happy with. I have the power to change myself and my life and feel happier with who I am.*

Locking into this experience of empowerment made Billy a fitness convert who showed up for every workout on tour and created his own system of fitness and trail running at home. He went from doing zero pull-ups to fifty per session. The rest of us watched his newfound self-assurance grow onstage, like he was stepping into a stronger version of himself who no longer held back what he had to show.

Though on the surface, the moral of the story is that anytime you can land a great job that'll give you a six pack you should take it, there's a deeper message here: Getting physically strong shifted how Billy felt about himself. Gaining control of his body made him feel more in control of his life. We all have a "stage" or an arena where we want to feel more confident. For some people it's work, for others it's relationships or their art. And even though we can write a hundred Post-it notes or try to think a thousand good thoughts about having more self-assurance, I think the route to it starts in the body. Confidence stems from a very visceral feeling that you deserve to be in your body and it's okay to take up space. Some people have it in spades — they just came in that way, or maybe their early circumstances were such that feeling like master of the universe is natural for them. But the rest of us have to build it, and then maintain it, and for that I turn to fitness first and foremost.

I spent a few years trying things the other

Exercise is like rocket fuel for your brain. It makes it easier to learn new things — a benefit I learned about from seminal fitness-as-brain-juice book *Spark* by John Ratey, PhD. As Dr. Ratey explains, exercise primes your brain for learning and puts you in a much better place to understand and remember things than if you'd stayed sedentary. Part of that is due to the secretion of something called BDNF, which stands for brain-derived neurotrophic factor. This special substance helps the neurons that make mental connections get stronger and protects them from dying. (The opposite is also true: staying sedentary leads to neural connections getting "pruned" — a neurological example of "use it or lose it.") This means that exercise is one of the best interventions you can do for your brain health at all stages of life, whether you're studying in school, hustling on the job, or wanting to stay sharp as you age. It doesn't take hours of effort to encourage BDNF to be released — twenty to forty minutes of even a moderately heart-pumping activity like brisk walking will trigger a significant surge.

way around: mustering false courage or trying to shadowbox my demons, talking them out of their negative stories. Those strategies worked to an extent. But the confidence always felt a little forced; it wasn't easy or graceful. I only got the real line on confidence when I built it from the core out by — literally — developing a stronger body with a solid center, grounded legs, and a more flexible, more capable spine. As the separate parts of my physicality began functioning as an integrated whole, my posture changed. I began standing taller. As I discovered my scapula — the muscles that hold your shoulders on the back of your body so they don't slump forward — and strengthened my back, my chest opened up and expanded. No more looking down or avoiding another's gaze; the way I carried myself changed. From that place came a shift in how I walked through the world. More open, more solid, less apologetic, more at ease. Though you might not notice it unless you compare my older music to new, my voice changed, too — a result, I think, of my diaphragm getting conditioned like any other muscle. I believe I sing better, with more range. Of course, performing with Faith helps me stretch myself, too. She's one hell of a singer to keep up with onstage.

As a performer, confidence makes or breaks

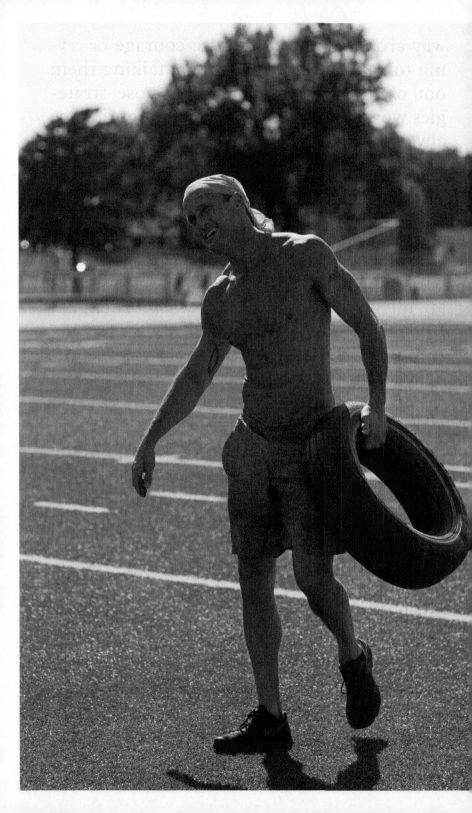

you. You have to know from the essence of your being that you have a worthwhile song to sing and a valuable story to tell. It's about the energy — you need to be able to really let it rip, without a doubting Thomas bumbling into your head, questioning what you're doing. But the same is true in any walk of life. Confidence isn't about looking like Jason Momoa or Beyoncé; it's the quality you develop that helps you say yes to new possibilities when you might otherwise say no; it's what makes other people feel safe to share their best selves with you or throw the pass your way, sure that you won't fumble. Confidence primes you for the opportunity that might knock once, and once only. Without confidence, you hesitate or choke, and then sometimes discover it's gone.

I heard a snippet of a wise-sounding writer talking on the radio. He said, "Change the way you *act* to change the way you *think;* don't try to change the way you *think* to change the way you *act.*" That was it in a nutshell: becoming the better you is easier when you start with the action that expresses what you want to feel. When you physically embody confidence, even if you don't believe you have it, you gain confidence. My band and I use this trick every night on tour in our pre-show ritual. We pace the halls backstage a little, rotating our shoulders open, releasing our necks. I flex my spine, breathe deep, and expand from the inside out. Sometimes I thump my chest a few times for good measure to get the blood flow going. If I feel anxiety, I've learned not to try to banish it but to rename it. It's excitement. Then I grab my version of my game jersey — my black cowboy hat — and go from Tim the dad, husband, and high school friend to Tim the musician and performer you showed up to see.

The good news is that getting fitter and stronger starts to make this happen naturally. Most types of shorter-duration exercise slightly raise testosterone, the hormone that both men and women need to feel empowered; strength training, especially "compound moves" using multiple joints (like weighted squats) boost it higher. (The surge of confidence-boosting testosterone is one reason you feel like a total rock star after a great strength training session.) When you develop a solid center through smart strength training and when you create flexibility in your body through mobility work, the way you hold yourself changes and even the way you sit changes — you're less restricted and you breathe deeper. It's like the scaffolding for a confident state of being has been installed within you. This makes you feel more comfortable and relaxed in yourself, which radiates outward for other people to feel. The more comfortable you are in yourself, the smoother relationships go, too. Who feels heard or seen when one person is posturing or talking all the time, trying to mask their inadequacy? And when you don't have such a tight hold on what you need to happen, more possibilities seem to come at you, as if you just created some space for them. You know how they say that success breeds confidence and confidence breeds success? That's exactly what happens by training the body to stand tall and strong; you retrain the brain to stop playing small. And it all starts from a pledge to pick up some free weights or do lunges across your lawn.

The next time you start to shrink into yourself, feel powerless, or lose faith in what you can be, please do me one favor: stretch your back wide, breathe deeply into your ribs, expand like a starfish — and tell your inner doubter to go to hell.

#5: You Feel Freedom, Connection, and Joy

I'm with one of my daughters in the deep blue void of the Caribbean waters near my family's home in the Bahamas, experiencing

111

the benefits of having trained for strength and agility for months before our trip: I'm touching a state of freedom and flow, and feeling at one with my world.

The ocean is my sanctuary; it's where I love to go to unplug from the buildup of everyday drama, to let noise fall to silence, and exhale any worries into bubbles that dance up to the light and then disappear. Sometimes it's where I relish alone time, some much-needed isolation. Other times it's where my kids and I play. In the ocean we can come back to ourselves if we've gotten pulled in too many directions or we're feeling fractured as a family. And if I've logged my hours working out on dry land, I get a true gift upon slipping into the water; the physical effort comes easily and for an hour or two, my mind drops fully into my body, totally present, as close to quiet as I get. It's as if my body performs all the physical functions required — kick, dive, spin — with zero supervision or direction. That lets my mind relax fully, get saturated in the majesty around me, and deeply enjoy. The sensation is almost overwhelming in its fullness: *I am not just* in *this beautiful world; I am* of *this world. I breathe into it, and it breathes into me.*

I don't take these moments of grace for

granted. They're precious because they're rare. All the trying and efforting stops for a moment, and the sensation is of being suspended in something bigger than myself. Just being there, afloat in azure water, is everything. It is enough. For a guy who's pretty relentless about working hard and achieving, and who didn't have many moments of pure peace as a kid, catching this feeling is priceless — a peak experience of feeling alive and connected; the X-factor feeling that I'm doing exactly what I'm supposed to be doing right now and nothing else matters but this. It's a sense of being at one with the world. There are many paths up the mountain to touch the peak; physical exertion and movement are what connect body, mind, and spirit for me.

But I've learned it doesn't come for free: that's why I try to get creative in the gym, on the field, and in the pool, working all kinds of challenging movements and ranges of motion so that when the chance comes to get out into nature and play, my condition is on point; I can slip into the moment and barely have to think about it.

My band's bassist, Paul, talks about running on the beach in similar way. He says it's his meditation and his song — a song he has to sing every day or two because when

Want an instant confidence boost? Just change the shape of your body. As Roger taught me, standing tall with your feet hip-width apart and raising your arms in a "V" above your head isn't called "Victory Pose" in yoga for nothing. That open-chested, sky-touching posture expands your body outward and upward, the exact configuration that researchers like social psychologist Amy Cuddy say can flip the switch to a state of empowerment. (Is it a coincidence that it's also the shape you're supposed to

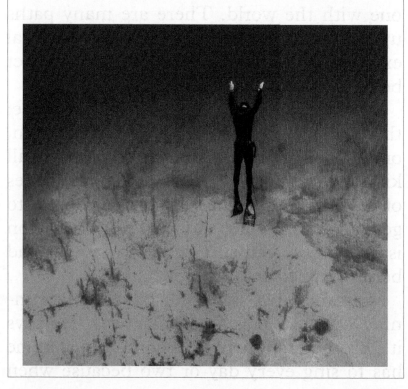

make to scare away a wild animal coming at you on a trail?) Try holding it for ten deep breaths, expanding your rib cage on each inhale and letting your breath travel to your fingertips. Meanwhile let the weight of your body root down into the ground through your heels. Don't overthink this. Just breathe, relax your face, take up some space, and notice how you feel after you're done.

he falls into his rhythm and hits his stride, moving through nature as free as a bird (or rangy Irish Wolfhound in his case), he feels cocooned in peace and happiness. It's how he reconnects to what's bigger than he is — earth and the elements and the liveliness of nature. And it's how he processes his feelings and makes sense of his life. When your body hits a rhythm by moving repetitively on a walk, run, or swim, the mind can fall into order and coherence. Instead of bombarding you with chatter, something else can enter, like flashes of insight or reflections about your life. It's like you can hear a wiser part of yourself speaking; you're connected to yourself more deeply.

115

Dean, our fiddle player, has discovered his own kind of connection from getting stronger and fitter. His limber, agile body, developed through regular training sessions, helps him keep up with his three active boys on Eagle Scout expeditions through forests and caves, or scrambling up and down perilous cliffs. Dean's hard work in the Gorilla Yard helps him bond with his family and experience his life fully, heart and soul.

One of our team's managers found another way to train her way to a peak experience. She hiked daily at a Nashville park wearing a loaded backpack so that she could fulfill her dream of a high Andes trek at twelve thousand feet. Getting in shape let her experience the high of exploring and adventuring on top of the world.

Moments like these are ours to claim; we all deserve them. They don't have to cost anything but time and effort. The clincher is putting in some of that effort up front, so you feel ready to take action and have the capacity to do so when the time arrives. When your body is strong and integrated, it's easy to enjoy a bike ride around the neighborhood or over rugged trails — or a horse ride for that matter. It feels good, not painful, to jog with your stroller by the river or carry your kid in a backpack through the park. You see no obstacles to a spontaneous ski or snowshoe through a magical winter landscape with a new friend — or taking a surf class at sunrise, if that's what calls your name. Everything that nature offers to let you feel free, awake, and alive becomes available to you when you've kept up your condition through exercise. So if you're unsure whether to get your gear on tomorrow, remember this: You get three prizes from paying into your health daily through training: You get a body capable of carrying you up hills and through valleys, across lakes and over desert tundra; the skills and strength to keep exploring well into your golden years; and something even more special, too. You get your own personal mainline into states that are always out there but can be hard to tap sometimes: joy, gratitude, and grace.

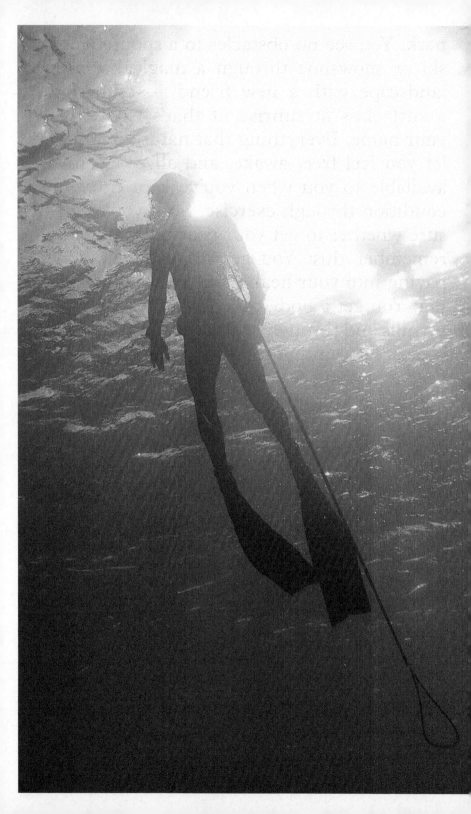

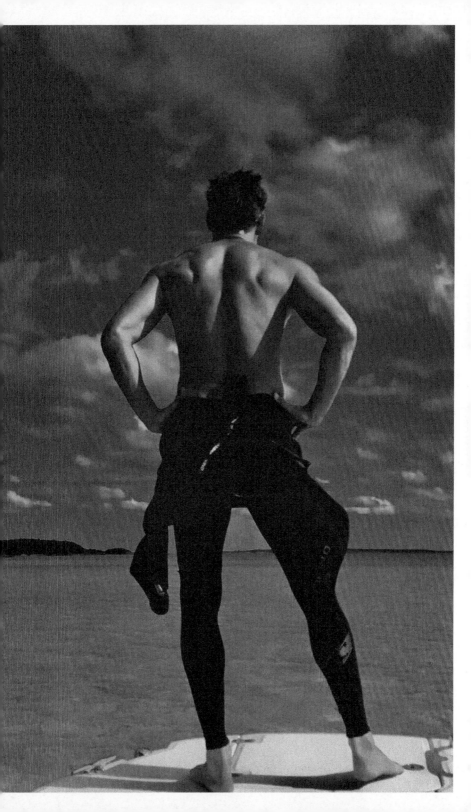

PART II
TRAIN THE MIND

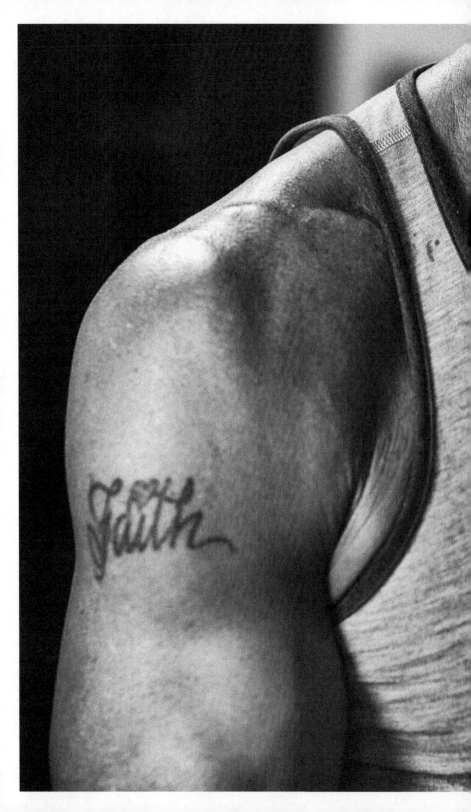

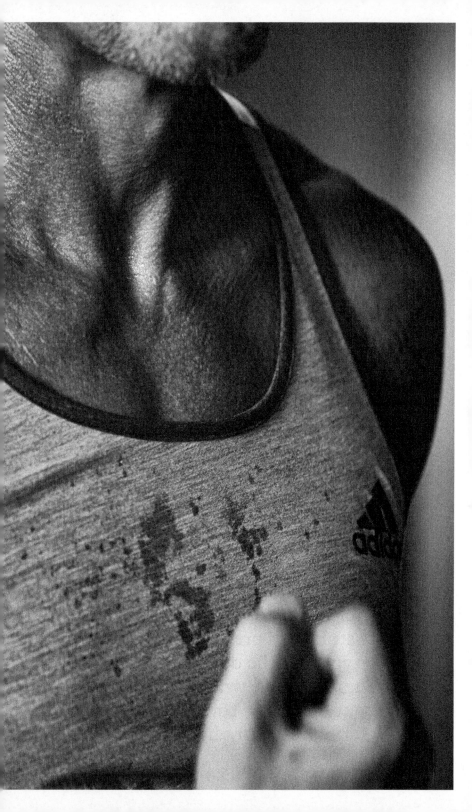

Come with me as I wander down from our house outside Nashville to the converted garage that is my home gym/man cave. It's nothing excessive by any means — about eight hundred feet all said and done — but inside, my most-used training gear is organized cleanly and clearly, and the space suits my needs just fine. There's a treadmill for loosening things up in the morning by walking then speed walking, varying the incline up and down. There's a rower for doing timed intervals during a conditioning workout. Naturally there are dumbbells racked in order from ten pounds up to sixty pounds, a family of kettlebells, and assorted barbell plates for lifting, jerking, pressing.

That stuff is all pretty standard, but what's not so typical is the design on the walls. The gym's mirrors and windows look like something out of a New York City subway in the '80s; scribbles of my handwriting, in thick white Sharpie pen, are scattered all over the glass haphazardly. Above the dumbbells, capital letters command *FOCUS*. By the boxing bag, the black writing urges *Fight!* And to the right of that a line exhorts, *Be Relentless!* It goes on: *Never underestimate your value* reads one slogan; *Lead with your Heart* reads another. *Always be prepared for your opportunity* counsels the northwest window, and *Be encouraging to my girls & build them up* counsels the mirror by the exit.

Motivational graffiti may not be Faith's idea of decor, but, luckily, I have full clearance to go rogue in this room. My tagging habit started as a way to help me switch gears mentally the minute I hit the gym. If you've ever been in the locker room of any sports team, you might have seen something similar — mottos taped onto locker doors and mantras inked boldly by coaches on the top of the team's whiteboards. The words act as a shortcut for the athletes to get to the peak state of concentration and effort. They remind them at a glance what they came here to do: Play the best game of their lives and strive through thick and thin to win.

My scribbles work the same way, though the primary reason is mundane, closer to a shopping list: I forget this stuff if I don't write it down. We all do! Our highest intentions and our most practical to-dos have a habit of floating away just seconds after they enter our minds.

The effect is more than just memory jogging. My Sharpie mantras act like anchors holding me accountable to the person I want to be. They cue me to remember that every workout starts in the mind with the attitude I bring to the gym, trail, or court. Because your mind-set determines the most important part of the health equation: whether you actually show up for it. I believe that 80 percent of getting in shape is knowing *why* you're working out and having strategies in place to support that *why*. The actual exercise only accounts for about 20 percent. So if you don't consider yourself athletic or you haven't developed skills on the mat, in the field, or in the pool, you're in luck. The most crucial piece of training is mental — and anyone can do it.

How smoothly the process of getting in shape goes is not determined by the number of sneakers in your closet or whether pull-ups come easy. There's no workout "type." It's more about your capacity for ownership and accountability, mental qualities that can be learned and honed as you go.

I recently learned that when researchers asked people how much they'd moved in a day and then tracked them physically, they found that almost everyone overestimated how much they exercised or how hard they pushed. The same discrepancy occurs between what we *say* we'll do — whether it's a New Year's resolution or just a plan to work out in the morning — and what we *actually* do. A lot of times there's quite a gap. It's just a fact of human nature: our default state is to conserve energy. After all, for most of human history, we've had to avoid expending energy unnecessarily in case the food runs out tomorrow. We're also partly wired to stay safe at all costs and cling to the familiar — to avoid the danger inherent in taking risks and trying new things. You could say that it's natural to want to hunker down and do less.

Except that we're living in unnatural times, in which food is always available and radically different from what it used to be, and we're not using our bodies all day long to take care of basic needs — it's like movement has been engineered out of our lives. So doing what feels "natural" is not gonna cut it. The truth is we need to *use* the excess energy we consume in our diet and find *more* ways to challenge bones, muscles, ligaments, and joints so they grow in strength and functionality.

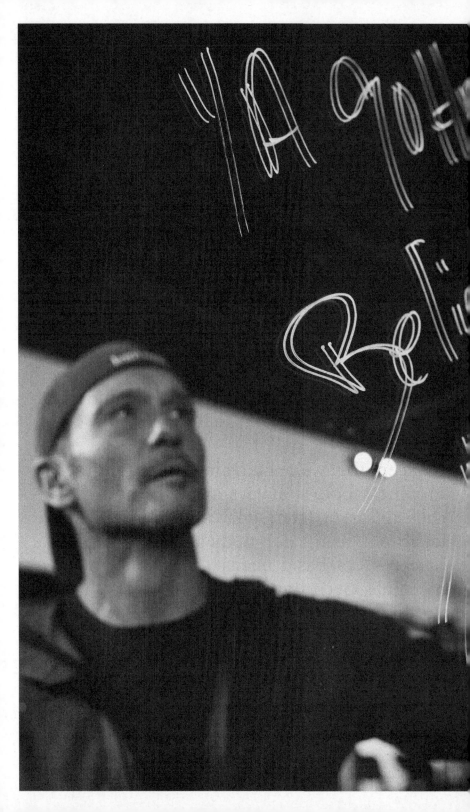

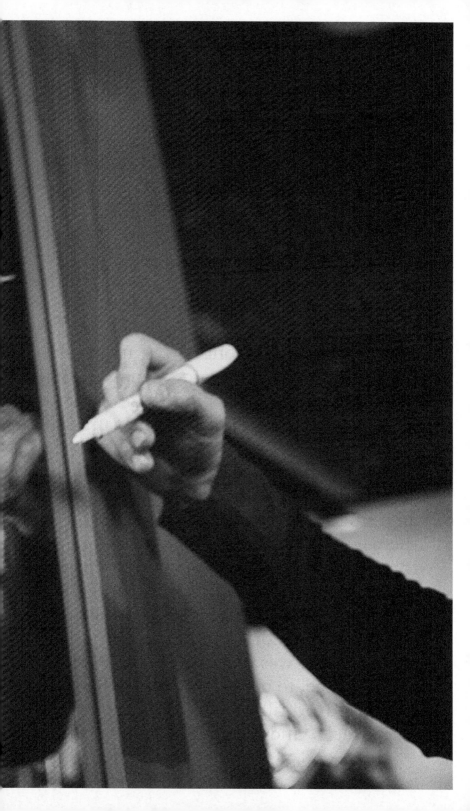

What's helped me override some of my reflexive impulses has been gaining an awareness of my mind and what it's telling me. Most notably: *I'll work out when I feel like it.* The problem is, there are plenty of times when I don't feel like it! I've learned that relying on being "in the mood" to work out is an unreliable way to operate. Let's face it, the perfect mood is always fickle — whether you're talking about health, love, or life. And good intentions aren't strong enough to get you out of your warm bed for a cold morning run. I've learned that my mind needs to follow something stronger: commitment.

It's often said that commitment is a quality that's falling out of fashion these days. Call it the fear of missing out, it's that unspoken attitude that something better might show up soon, or what you choose might be disappointing, so you don't want to go all in on anything just yet. But I'm not certain that's the whole truth. Most everyone is following through on some kind of commitment every day. I had to remember that when I hit my turning point a few years back. I was undisciplined and ignoring my body, but I wasn't a lost cause! I was committed to my work, to my marriage, to my kids. After all, Faith and I never waited till we "felt like" taking Maggie, Gracie, and Audrey to school; we just did it regardless. We didn't decide "in the moment" whether we felt like getting groceries or making dinner — we'd committed to feeding the family in advance. The trick was to take that same level of commitment I had to others and transfer it over to my own body and health.

Commitment is the bridge that links ideas and action, helping you to cross the divide between dreaming about something and actually achieving it. You need it solidly in place to live a healthy lifestyle, because anytime your goal tests your physical capability or asks you to put off gratifying your desire for comfort, the impulsive side of your mind will come up with lots of compelling reasons to quit.

The Three Ds of Commitment

Though I wasn't necessarily conscious of it at the time, looking back on it now I recognize that there were three main qualities to getting my head in the game and fully committed to a fitness routine. I call them the Three Ds: drive, discipline, and deep focus. They're the keys to making your mind become your ally in this process, helping you to get traction on healthy habits in the first place and then helping to make them last. I like to imagine the three Ds as three

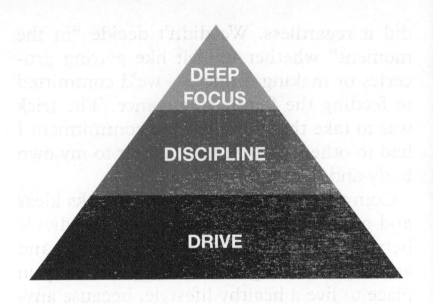

layers of a solid pyramid of commitment.

Let's look at the first layer: *Drive* is the foundation of our pyramid; it has to be there for the whole thing to work. Drive is your motivation, your inner force that compels you to act. *Discipline* is the middle layer; it's how you develop and deploy the strategies to ensure you take action. Ever heard the saying "Failing to prepare is preparing to fail"? Discipline gets you prepared enough that you walk the walk and don't just talk the talk. *Deep focus* is the top of the pyramid, the apex. You can explore it once discipline is firmly in place. Deep focus is the ability to drop into a zone of no distraction so when you're working out, you're fully present to it, putting in effort and reaping maximum benefits. Some people also refer to it as *flow*.

The cool thing about this stack of skills is that they are applicable across all of your life — they're not just effective for your workouts. When you master this pyramid, you gain an even bigger prize than a better state of health. You train your mind to be your friend — the kind of friend who cheers you on and keeps you focused on your goals instead of tempting you away from them and sabotaging your efforts.

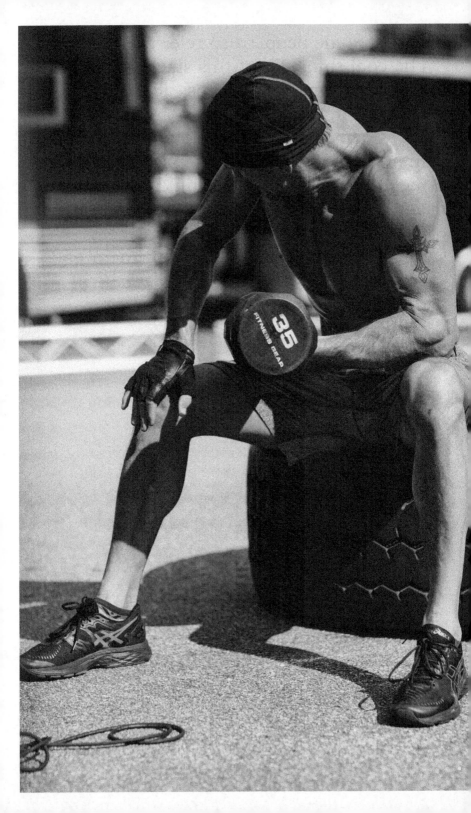

CHAPTER 3
DRIVE

Creating something — anything — asks you to draw from a deep place. Whether it's a song, a relationship, or a healthier lifestyle, if creation were simply a matter of checking off some boxes, we'd all be cruising down easy street, fit as fiddles and happy as can be. But that would also take the miracle out of it. Anything truly meaningful comes from a kind of effort that demands looking past the surface and sometimes wrangling with what you find in the murky depths. That is why the first part of our fitness formula is mastering your mind.

Commitment is the bridge that links ideas and action, helping you to cross the divide between dreaming about something and actually achieving it. You need it solidly in place to live a healthy lifestyle, because anytime your goal tests your physical capability or asks you to put off gratifying your desire for comfort, the impulsive side of your mind will come up with lots of compelling reasons to quit.

It's often said that in order to move toward a better version of yourself, you need to be powered by the charge of a big, important *why*. You need to be clear on the value of your work and feel excited about the goal you're working toward — especially when you're starting a process that will be tough at times and that will test your edges. You're gonna want to know, *What do I get out of this? What will it mean in the long run?* That's where identifying and cultivating your drive comes in. Drive is the force of all your "whys" put together. If you can tap into your drive before taking action, your efforts will be more focused and stronger, and more likely to reach their target.

We don't all come into this world with the same inherent level of drive. Maybe I have more of it than average because intensity is in my DNA. The force of urgency to create has been hardwired in me from the get-go: Intensity manifests in the music I make and the shows I do. It's the intensity a lot of artists feel: an urge to make sense of their story, turn life's sour lemons into sweeter lemonade, and put some part of themselves out there to reach and connect with others. Intensity for me is the desire to feel the fear and do it anyway. My artistic whys tend to stare me in the face at all times, prodding me to take chances.

Despite that fact that I'm regularly engaged with this kind of creative risk-taking, when it came time to turn things around physically, it required a lot of effort — and still does! I had to put my motivation for building health under the magnifying glass, identify it clearly, then catch it and give it some love. Because motivation is like inspiration — it can be elusive. It'll show up for a while — like on a perfectly sunny spring morning when the air is fresh and swimsuit season's around the corner — then just like that, it'll disappear. Once I got the whys wrangled and harnessed, however, it was game on. My whys inspired me to go cold turkey on my vices and helped me get to the place where I can count the number of days I've skipped workouts or stopped halfway through on one hand. Now that I'm getting older and wiser, it's also helping me temper my pace so I don't burn out — but that's my particular lesson to learn.

The takeaway I want to share is that staying superconnected to my whys has proven to be a primary ingredient in my special sauce of health. I've learned to prize the feeling of wanting something badly and to feed the flames of it deliberately. Because you can't expect to feel your drive pulsing through your veins at all times, especially today when distractions come knocking. Have you ever felt like your mind is pitching you anything else to do *but* exercise, just when you're about to gear up to sweat? It'll say, *Check the news; look up the weather in Boise or Billings, check your e-mail one last time.* Or it says, *Hold up, you better check in with the kids, then do that chore you dropped yesterday* — totally reasonable-sounding stuff that nevertheless puts a kibosh on your plans.

Connecting to your drive and then tending to it daily is a way to reinforce your mind against all that background noise. When you're about to lose your momentum, your drive is the giant billboard in front of your face emblazoned with a supersized message in Technicolor. *Hey, dummy, this is why you're doing it — remember?*

The way I see it, there are two components to drive. There are your rational whys, the good reasons for taking care of your body that anyone would agree make sense. Then there is your nonrational, deeply personal why — your private passion about how you want to feel and who you want to be. It's like one part head and one part heart. To successfully stay motivated, it's good to get clear on both: to consider your reason and activate your passion and give each of them the best seats in the house so you don't lose sight of them. Let's take a closer look at how that works.

Reason: Drive's Smart and Predictable Side

Reason is the good-sense side of motivation; the logic for working out and dialing up your health habits. Your reasons are the things you would say out loud and not feel shy about. Logical reasons are different from person to person, but they tend to be centered around what is technically known as "extrinsic motivation" — meaning that they are shaped by external voices and rewards. For example, a rational why might be a doctor's advice (or her ultimatum!), a desire to look better to change how you're perceived, or even a need to be capable and available for others. Many personal trainers say that these extrinsic motivations are the reasons their clients walk in the door; they matter, and they can certainly keep you showing up at the trailhead or the gym.

My primary reason is clear: I've made my job an athletic job. My fitness has become core to how I perform and who I am, and I know it's part of why things are going pretty

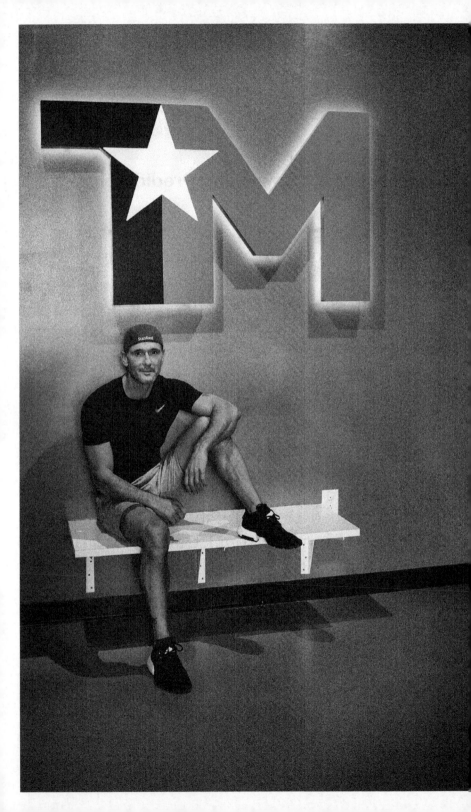

well with my career today. For me it's entirely logical: if a pro football player trains eight to nine months a year to play at the top of his game, so must I. Second, I want to set a good leadership role for everyone around me. If I keep it rolling, it's likely they will, too. Then there's an extrinsic motivation that is very external: I like fitting into my clothes! I've landed on what works for me, and I'd rather work hard to keep it that way than have to adjust the formula.

When Faith kicked her fitness into a new level for our Soul2Soul tour, she had her own solid reason. After taking a hiatus from touring to focus on fulfilling her dream of mothering — a calling she embodies with amazing love and grace — she wanted to be able to perform the way her heart guided her to perform: with everything she's got. If you've ever seen Faith up there under the lights, you know how physical she is — she dances all over that stage! Her primary reason for dialing up her workouts was to get to her personal level of "tour shape." Her drive propels her to run the stadium steps alongside me. I love seeing that side of my wife.

The members of our touring road family have their own reasons. For guitarist Denny, it was to counteract the sedentary and — to his refined senses — the relatively high toxic load of the touring and traveling lifestyle. For bassist Paul, it was to make sure the *Groundhog Day* effect of being on tour didn't drive him to "make the wrong kind of fun." But there are many other reasons that maybe you relate to:

You want to manage stress or anxiety on an everyday basis, so it never gets a jump on you or dictates how you react.

Your doctor has suggested that you get your weight or cholesterol under control to avoid developing health complications.

You'd like to go down a clothing size or two (or more) or look leaner, curvier, or more developed and defined.

You hope to stay mobile and functional as you get older and maintain your independence from others, so your kids don't have to take care of you.

It's important to you to model a healthy lifestyle for your family and get all of you on a good path.

Or maybe it's more specific athletic goals that drive your reason, such as learning how to ski or scuba dive or play tennis or golf or just getting your body primed enough to go hard and have lots of fun. Maybe your good reason is even a godly one: you believe your body is your temple, and you glorify God through taking care of it well. There are probably a hundred other reasons you could come up with and all would be sound ones. They'll help push your ship off the dock and may sustain you to solid results. But in my experience, the rational thinking alone doesn't fully cut it. If it did, we'd all be much fitter, physically and mentally — after all, the logical information about the health benefits of exercise have been well publicized for years, and as that earlier study showed, most of the population still isn't moving their bodies nearly enough.

I firmly believe that to stick out this gig you have to turn things up a notch and set logic on fire. You have to find that part of you that wants to achieve your goals so badly it burns a little. To do that you have to connect to something wilder than reason — your personal passion. Remember the part of the TRUMAV credo that says, "dream big . . . envision the future . . . answer to something greater"? Those words are passion speaking.

Passion: Drive's Wild and Thrilling Side

Passion is the sense of purpose that stirs you up inside. It's reason's rogue cousin — it's irrational and likes to go out of bounds. Passion is emotional not logical. It comes from the heart.

143

Have you ever been pounding the final stages of a run, carried on air by a rousing anthem in your earbuds, and imagined yourself crossing an imaginary finish line with crowds cheering at your triumph? Hit your rhythm biking up a hill and felt like the yellow-jersey pack leader of the Tour de France? Or found your groove skiing downhill and felt like Lindsey Vonn on her gold-medal run as the wind whistled in your ears? Or, if you haven't been active for a while, have you felt that surge of *Wow-how-cool-is-that* awe when you watch the Olympics or attend a pro sporting event? That rush of excitement you feel *when movement moves you* is your passion speaking to you. It ignites the urge to reach far and finish strong. It tells you that going big is your destiny just like anyone else's and that glowing skin, bright eyes, and defined muscles are already in you; you just have to find them.

The technical term for passion is *intrinsic motivation*: the desire to take action that is fully your own because it scratches an itch *only you know.* You might call it your inspiration or your higher self speaking. I like to call it your maverick self — it's the aspect of you that feels the fire to claim a bigger and brighter life. The you that burns with the desire for change and that has the capacity to be a leader — a warrior, even. It sees the bird's-eye view of where you could take your life if you didn't create limits, and it tries to set you on that course. Let's not get trapped by logic here: The maverick you feels like anything is possible. I won't go as far to say it's the *best* you that exists — that's a lot of pressure. But it's definitely the *better* you, the one who takes risks, grows, and accomplishes new things, and for flashes of time gets to feel invincible. When our bassist Paul, who's in his fifties, leaps into the air doing splits onstage like Flea from the Red Hot Chili Peppers, I always get a smile on my face: That's his inner maverick letting loose.

My fitness journey reminded me to listen when my passion speaks. When I felt the wild rush to take my training to the next level and get in the best shape of my life, I heard it saying, *"You've come this far, son, why not take it all the way?"* And I enjoyed that rush. It made me feel like a kid again playing at Superman, imagining that I had it in me to leap buildings and soar through space. That's why I didn't shoo the sensation away. I entertained it because one of my passions is testing my limits and finding out how far I can go. Some people probably thought I was a little crazy — just as they may think *you're* a little crazy if you follow your passion. I say you're crazy not to.

Because the urge to push yourself and be bigger exists as your guide; it's there to prompt you to shake things up, do something differently, and unleash your potential. A good example of this is my younger sister Sandy, who took ownership of her health after years of ups and downs. Her initial why was logical: she was starting to experience health complications from being overweight, and she wanted to turn around her health for herself and her kids. But privately her passion spoke, too. It said, *I'm sick of feeling tired and out of shape! I want to let the real me out now, the one that's been covered up for way too long.* She knew this would involve a deep personal journey, one that had her reckon with our childhood and our past and her feelings about who she was and what she wanted. Sandy bravely did that inner work and fearlessly seized hold of passion to drive the actions that created a whole new reality for herself. It hasn't always been easy for Sandy, but her results have been awesome. To me, she embodies not only the idea of drive but also grit and no small amount of grace, as she inspires others in her family and community to do the effortful thing, too.

Listening to the whispers from this bigger, bolder, invincible you breathes positivity and potential into your current reality, lifting you higher and giving you hope. It reminds you of what you know you could do and be even if you're not doing or being that yet, waking up your sense of confidence. In fact, when I decided early on to turn my life around through six weeks of daily exercise, I was listening to a private passion that I haven't told many people about, but that helped reinforce my commitment to dialing in a cleaner, sharper lifestyle: The desire to become a pilot. What does flying a plane have to do with working out? you might ask. Surely it only requires sitting in a seat, learning technical skills? Well, I had always wanted to fly a plane. I fly frequently for work and often talked to the pilots of our planes, asking them questions about their scariest moments and challenges, watching the process of landing and wondering if I could do it myself one day. I felt called to master the challenge of guiding a plane, much like I'd learned how to explore underwater, a hobby that allows me to feel completely capable and free. But I knew that flying would require being 200 percent on point with all my mental muscles fully honed. There's no room for error when you're thousands of feet up. And that aligned perfectly with my goal of cleaning out all cobwebs, getting laser focused, and performing at a high level of integrity. So I harnessed this passion and used it to drive myself in my fitness goals: I made finding a flight instructor my pot-of-gold reward at the end of the rainbow. I told myself that if I turned my health around, I'd be primed to get in the cockpit. It was another way of testing myself to see just how far I could go.

Looking back at my process of coming out of the darkness and into the light, I see how life-saving it was to listen to my passion. The effort required for flight training kept me hooked into lifestyle goals at all times. To study and practice the art and science of flight, I had to stay totally alert physically and mentally. It retrained my brain to find rewards in difficult but positive things and overwrote some of the old stories that can play on loop in my mind during moments of stress, like the one that goes, *You didn't even finish college, what do you know about science, or business, or flying planes?* Well, hell: Maybe I didn't finish college, but now I was aviating with total precision! The more I perfected the skills required, the more accomplished I felt about every aspect of myself and the more my "upward cycle" of healthy living got powerfully reinforced.

EMBODY THE IDENTITY

Arnold Schwarzenegger is purported to have said, when discussing how he turned himself from army recruit to bodybuilding champion, "Create a vision of who you want to be, then live into that picture as if it were already true." In a nutshell: Imagine yourself as an active, agile, energized person — viscerally picture and feel yourself as an impassioned athlete, a dedicated yogi, an up-for-it outdoorsman or woman, or simply a person who communes with nature on a daily walk. Imagine how it feels to be them, how it looks to be them, how you move when you're them. If it feels awkward to tap into a completely unknown version of yourself, see if you have a memory of yourself at your peak, on your best day ever, or a phase of life when you crushed it. Then click into that "peak identity" to take a step in the right direction to reach your health goals. Ask, "What action would that other 'me' take right now — go back to bed or get up and salute the sun? Stay inside from the rain or put on the slicker and get running? Check Twitter at the dog park or do lunges and squats while Fido's playing?"

It's called embodying the identity you want to be. Just like throwing up your arms into a victory pose as you cross an imaginary finish line on your gym treadmill promotes the physiology of empowerment, embodying the qualities you want is not just fantasy play — it's part of a proven strategy for supporting yourself to make choices that are aligned with your higher goals.

And it's a useful trick for taking your small self out of the equation with all his or her engrained habits and actions, and jumping straight to the better choice that will get you closer to where you want to go. Remember the motto *Change the way you act to change the way you think?* This hack is basically your grandma schooling you with common sense: to get in the mood for something, don't wait for the mood to arrive. Start doing the something and let it create the mood.

YES YOU CAN

In the book *Reinventing Yourself,* author Steve Chandler offers a useful tool for conditioning your mind. Anytime you admire a feat that someone else can do, practice saying, "I can do that, too!" Too often we say things like "I could never do that," which seems like it's humility speaking, but is actually your cautious or limiting self telling your brain it will never happen. The simple phrase reinforces the idea of yourself as less capable or stuck. Saying out loud "I can do that — if I train, practice, and work hard" starts to lay down a different and more positive track for your mind to run on. "I can" repeated enough times retrains the brain if it's been hearing "I can't" for some time. And it's a generous way to think: You're seeing the gifts in others and seeing them inside yourself, too.

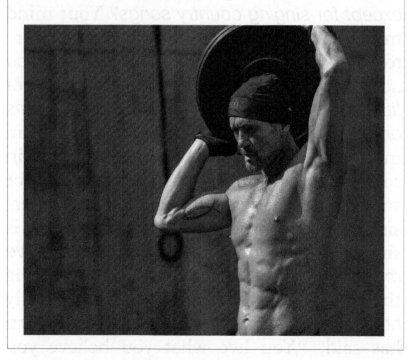

I don't mean to suggest that stoking the flames of passion is always easy. the burning desire to feel better can be hard to ignite if life's rained on you a little or if disappointment and hurt have clouded your hope. Dreams don't sprout well in soggy ground, and old stories that got engraved into your mind early on, often through no fault of your own, can be hard to root out. The mind likes to cling to what it knows and what feels familiar — even if it's a way of thinking about yourself that doesn't serve you anymore. Like my own old standard tune: *You didn't even stick with college, Tim, what do you know except for singing country songs?* Your mind might play a similar refrain should you dare to reach for healthy: *You're not athletic; you don't have the body for it; you're too old to get fit. People like you don't join boutique gyms or feel welcome in fitness tribes.* Take it from me: We're all shadowed by those voices in some shape or form, just sometimes and for some of us they yell louder and more persistently than others. Even if your voice is simply saying, *I don't have it in me to move my body today,* it's a limiting belief impeding the action that, if you did it, would actually *help* you have energy. Many a self-help guru has said, "You live what you believe you are." Limiting beliefs will derail you before you realize it's happening; they convince you to settle, even if what you're settling for isn't what you want. And when low self-worth gets a lock on you, it can chip away at your morale and energy and lead to apathy and poor choices, which in turn can make you feel so bad you make more poor choices — as I discovered at my lowest.

It's important to recognize that limiting voices don't tell the truth. Everyone "has the body" for enjoying moving at some level — whether it starts with lying down and breathing deeply or with lung-burning uphill sprints. Nobody's too old to move in some kind of way that feels good, and each person has the right to explore whatever experience of fitness they like.

When your passion feels half-buried under ash and extra-challenging to locate, it's a cue to try harder to connect with it — to find even just one ember. Because without passion, it's a lot harder to quit making the choices the old you has always made — like grabbing the doughnut instead of the grapefruit; taking the elevator instead of the stairs; getting all tangled up in the wrong kind of influence — and claim the choices the better you wants to make. The key in these instances is to have some self-compassion. Doubting,

If you've been struggling with or unhappy about your weight, you might find your mind telling you that getting fit will be more challenging for you than others. Reframe that limiting belief: One of my favorite maverick trainers, Adam Ticknor, likes to say it's easier to help a larger person get fit than a very skinny one. Why? You're already strong because you've been conditioned by carrying weight on your bones and joints; your posture is probably better than average because if you slump you feel the tension more acutely and correct it sooner; and you likely are more familiar with moving through discomfort, so your mind is already stronger in this regard. None of this is to make light of the mental and physical effort required to make change, but it can help to look at a situation through a new set of lenses. You might be further ahead than you think you are.

limiting voices will never get eradicated completely. It's part of being human; we're all a little broken, and life puts scratches on the record that will cause it to skip. That's especially the case if you've experienced any type of trauma, big or small, in your past. The scratches can feel quite deep. But that doesn't mean you're beholden to them. When the undermining voices start to pull you off course, take action, because keeping that spark of passion alive is essential to owning your health. There are a lot of ways to do this, but here are four of my go-to strategies for pushing back on the limiting thoughts that can subvert or sabotage your drive:

1 BECOME AWARE. When you hear yourself repeating an old script about your lack of talents, imperfect body, or low capability, tell it you recognize it for what it is — an old story that has no real bearing on who you actually are — and ask it to go take a hike. *You* run this show, and you're not beholden to old stories. Tame those tigers by turning your attention firmly to what you want to achieve, and keep them in their place.

2 CLEAR THE TENSION. There's a meaningful three-part exercise called "clearing" that Roger likes to teach as the prelude to moving and working out. We use it to release feelings that get in the way of change on a mental and

emotional level as well as a way to get energy, oxygen, and circulation moving in the body. This isn't as soft as it may seem — Roger trains movie assassins for a living, after all. What he knows is that the body is a storehouse of emotions. It will hold on to stress responses from daily life, as well as judgment, blame, or shame about your body or your failure to take care of it. That's because when we don't want to feel something difficult, we often contract physically, literally "stuffing things away" as physical tension held in our muscles and connective tissues. If we don't release it, the tension can change the way our muscles, tendons, and ligaments sit in the body, tightening the breath, causing restrictions, and even pulling the spine out of alignment. The result can be that it doesn't feel comfortable to be in your body or it just doesn't feel good to be you, which makes it even harder to get enthusiastic about exercising. Guess what? Even if you don't think you've judged, blamed, or shamed yourself lately, you're probably holding tension. It's what we do as sensitive beings — we take in stress from every corner just by merely having our eyes and ears open to life.

Roger believes the first step in any workout practice and for any body — whether you're a martial-arts stunt co-ordinator like him or more of an average joe — is to release tension and return to neutral. He calls it "clearing what's in the way" so that you can start from an unrestricted place with more space and freedom in body and mind. Clearing involves accepting yourself, forgiving yourself, and releasing the tension from the past. It can also mean releasing the tension patterns you've taken on from years of repetitive training, or overdoing one kind of activity — something he's familiar with from his years as a competitive fighter — so that the muscles are better able to adopt natural movement patterns like full squats. You can do one step, two steps, or all three, and you can return to these steps anytime you're feeling tired, unmotivated, or in need of a recovery moment after a long day or a boost to motivation or energy.

STEP 1: BREATHE. See the instructions for active breathing on page 97. Do at least two minutes of this breath pattern, releasing tension anywhere you detect it in the body.

157

STEP 2: RELEASE TENSION. Foam rollers and therapy balls are great tools for releasing tension and helping even the most hardheaded person get to a place of surrender and relaxation. They're designed to be used on the floor by placing them under the spine, hips, glutes, shoulders, rib cage, and legs to help you iron out tough kinks in your body — the places where tissues are stiff or stuck. Rolling also boosts lymphatic circulation, which helps carry toxins out of the body and boosts your immune system. Rolling out tension helps your body return to a "neutral" place without all the accumulated tension holding you back; for harried desk workers or elite athletes alike, Roger suggests regular sessions of rolling areas of the body from foot to skull, breathing fully as you go.

There are scores of foam rolling and therapy ball and massage ball videos online showing moves for various parts of the body. Lacrosse balls and softballs are also often used, carefully, under supertight spots like shoulders or deep in the muscles of your rear end; you nudge your weight onto them, breathe, and let the ball help create release. (Try to keep the ball pushing into denser muscles, tendons, and ligaments, not soft tissues, organs, and glands.) Rolling may not feel like "exercise" as you know it, but prepare to be surprised: You can do more for yourself in a few minutes of releasing tension, if that's what your body needs, than forcing yourself to lift heavy weights or sweat profusely. Roger likes to say that a rollout improves your functionality, longevity, agility, and pliability. After it, your muscles are free to move again naturally — you get closer to a clean slate. Depending on how vigorously you use them, these tools can help you de-stress and unwind before sleep or energize yourself when you're dragging. You can do a quick rollout of tight spots in two minutes, or take up to twenty minutes to work your whole body, head to toe and front and back.

STEP 3: PRACTICE ACCEPTANCE. It's not just physical muscles that get bound in restrictions. The mental ones do, too. When low self-worth is a sticking point getting in the way of being active, Roger suggests a reset. Look at your face in the mirror and take in your reflection. Be sure to breathe — chances are, you're holding your breath. Look deeply and notice what comes up as you take in the look of your skin, eyes, and hair; your frown lines or your laughter lines; the places that show excess stress and excess food or point to a lack of sleep, water, or joy. If you feel uncomfortable or you don't like what you see, he advises: Forgive all of it. Breathe (again). Let go of any blame. Release judgment of all the times you didn't work out or made a poor choice or drifted away from the person you want to be. Stay with this for a minute or two. Using the deliberate deep breaths described earlier, breathe in, release; breathe out, let go. Sure, it might be uncomfortable, but if you're working toward getting strong, discomfort can't faze you. The goal is to get to a place where you can say, without restriction, "I accept where I am today. I will start from here."

I'm not big on looking back. I tend to look forward, to focus on tomorrow. To my mind, forgiveness and letting go doesn't mean you suddenly have to love yourself; it's just about accepting that you are a work in progress, not a finished product. Acceptance is a neutral state; an acknowledgment that this moment is all that matters right now. That's a good place from which to start any health journey. And if it feels uncomfortable to allow something so neutral and simple where you usually feel angst, try this: Embrace the universal law of "Give and you shall receive." Your only job is to give some effort to the goal of owning your health. Even if you don't know how, why, or when the benefits will appear, trust that something good will come from it.

3 PUT THE NEGATIVITY TO WORK FOR YOU. I don't run away from fear of failure. I harness it, because there's power there. The friction created by wanting to do my best but fearing that I won't has a charge to it. It's taken me years to embrace, but now I lean into it when it arises. I'm a worrier who tends to lie in bed at night running through all the ways I've failed that day. Yet I've discovered that under that anxious energy lies the urge to make tomorrow even better, so I tap into *that* fire. The fear of mediocrity or of letting others down becomes the fuel to rise like a phoenix from the ashes of a rough day. And, after making that connection, I can usually fall asleep. Any artist knows that a little fear nipping at your heels keeps you on your toes. The trick is keeping the fear in its place: put most of your attention on the success you are creating, and only a sliver of it on the failure you want to dodge. Practices like this help you cultivate what psychologists call a growth mind-set, which is when you recognize that failure is part of progress and challenges are par for the course, and neither of them a reflection of who you truly are. You recognize that obstacles are real but know that they are temporary, and that you can overcome them.

4 **DITCH NEGATIVE VOICES.** Most important, even if none of these strategies feel possible to you, Outrun the voices and leave them in the dust! Sabotaging inner voices are slow and awkward companions. When you get moving and create a higher state of energy in your body, they can't keep up. The positive cascade of natural chemicals your body makes when you move, stretch, hurl, and sweat, not to mention the feeling of achievement that lifts your wings because of it, creates a much more convincing reality than any messages from the past that may be scrolling through your mind. And when

the flush of effort you generate inside burns off some of that fog, you might feel flashes of the passion that had been obscured.

I've got my own take on why sometimes it feels challenging to allow a better vision of yourself to come into focus. I think that some part of you knows that if you make contact with that maverick inside and let yourself truly feel your desire for better, some significant change could be required. If you start to have more energy, see more clearly, and feel more confident, then you'll *really* be accountable about where you choose to put your attention, time, and efforts. That could mean not only working out consistently but also changing how you eat, who you hang out with, how you show up for other people — maybe even what you do for work. I say, *don't let the fear of change fool you either.* That's just another limiting voice telling you that the better future you can't predict is scarier than the unsatisfying present you're in right now. You don't know what the future brings, you only know today! In the chapters to follow, I'll share some strategies that make the upgrade easier — from finding community to cooking clean food. For now, outwit that impulse to quit, expand your vision of yourself as large as it'll go, and know that with some ground lines in place, getting there won't be as hard as you think.

FINDING YOUR DRIVE

Are you ready to build the first layer in your pyramid of commitment? Grab a pen. Seriously — we're going back to basics here. Writing down goals clearly is actually a peak performance trick used by many a champion and trophy winner. Doing this helps you mentally "seal" your goals and dreams into your awareness, bringing your drive closer to the surface, where you can see it. It makes you more likely to remember your personal call to arms and primes you to feel excited, motivated, and confident to pursue your goals.

STEP 1 Write down three reasonable "whys" for establishing a regular fitness practice and keeping it up. These are your extrinsic, rational "whys." Keep it brief and to the point.

STEP 2 Next, turn up the heat to locate a passion for the practice. Remember, you want to want it badly because intensity helps drive you to action. Start by taking a big breath. Did you know that the word inspire literally means, "breathe in"? When you're inspiring yourself to play bigger, it's a good idea to expand your rib cage and feed more oxygen to your brain. Don't hold back — this information is for your eyes only.

Look at your reasons why and ask, *How does each of those reasons make me* feel — *what's the* feeling *behind why I want this to happen? What's the desire?* It might be a desire for energy, a desire to not hurt so much, a desire to not be scared about your health. Make that into an "I want" statement, preferably, "I want to feel _____." Feel how that feels; breathe into it, sit with it, and notice what else comes up. Write that down, too.

STEP 3 Now go bigger still. You're going to tap into your inner maverick by asking yourself a few questions. Start by asking, *When in the past have I felt most strong, fit, confident, emboldened, and proud of my body? What do I remember about how that felt and what it looked like?* The trick is not to approach this using your head, but listen to your heart and senses. If resistance bubbles up, note it but don't feed it. Come back to the vision. Imagine how this better version of you feels, stands, moves, and approaches the world — and how the world approaches this person. You don't have to write an essay here; a few words or phrases work fine. Jot them down the first things that come up.

If you're having trouble with this exercise, think of a moment when you've seen someone perform physically at a high level and felt a rush: *I want to move like that, I want to function like that, I want to look like that.* What would it look and feel like, to be that person? You could also think of your personal heroes. What qualities do or did they embody that you'd like to have? I'm inspired by people like George Washington and Winston Churchill — men who were great leaders and made brave choices. See what words or phrases come to mind.

Using either of these exercises, make what you discovered into an "I am" statement, preferably with two to three adjectives or nouns. "I am _____ x, y, and z."

Got that piece of paper? If it's messy, no problem. The point is to have this in writing. Put it somewhere you'll be able to see it or turn to it easily in your first few weeks of working out regularly.

Once you've connected with your personal "whys," don't get slack and let them fade into the background. Motivation is quick to show up but even faster to fade away. So you have to use some tricks to keep it top of mind. Here are the ones I've come to rely on most often.

Motivational Mantras

Even if you don't have gym mirrors to scribble on, you can make key words or phrases easily visible as you move through your day — from your bathroom mirror to your computer password to the refrigerator door. Take the words you jotted down above and build them out into phrases or mottos that are meaningful to you. Ask what your inner maverick's personal slogan would be, or think of a song lyric that nails the feeling your passion embodies. Have fun with it — movie titles, rallying cries, famous quotes, or just single words bolded and underlined like some of mine all count. If pictures work better for you than words, make it a visual exercise. Take screenshots of images that represent how you want to feel, or find an image of the heroes you identified and use them as quick reminders. They could be your home screen on a computer or phone, the cover of a journal, or (why not?) get them printed on a T-shirt!

Turn Up the Music

Nothing gets you over mental hurdles like a great track that lights you up from inside. I get fired up when the artist or band I'm listening to has it all — the song's well written, the way the track is produced is perfect, and the way they present themselves is cool. It makes me want to work harder as an artist, and my inner maverick starts to champ at the bit. The actual tunes I play might surprise you; it might be the Eagles one day or Bruno Mars the next. What matters is that you do you. Finding a playlist that connects you to your passion can help get you out of the starting blocks and scorching down the track, and inspire the impetus to give your final reps more guts than the first ones.

Track Your Results with 8 Questions

Train yourself to notice the positive outcomes of your efforts, no matter how small. Seeing results is the one of the most essential parts of accomplishing any goal. To do this, you have to practice looking at the subtle stuff, because the results of the good habits usually aren't as overt or seductive as the bad ones — the kind that change your state dramatically and give you undeniable hits and rushes of instant gratification. (That's why the negative habits get so addicting. Their effects are as in-your-face as a roller-coaster ride.)

One of the best ways to do this is to ask yourself the 8 questions on page 170–171 every time you exercise — and I mean every time, especially at first, when your practice might be fairly modest. Keep them on a piece of paper that you can glance at the end of your workout. The questions help you notice the small shifts that occur when

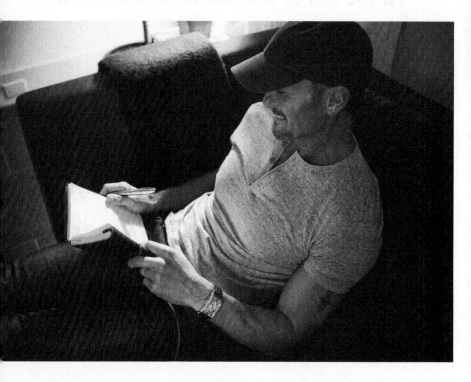

you exercise. They train your brain to feel the pleasure of reward and seek out *more* rewards gained the same way. Acknowledging positive results is one of the most powerful methods available to overwrite bad habits with good ones, because results give you gratification, and true gratification is a driver of habit formation. Your brain starts to light up at the thought of the workout, making it more compelling than other choices you could make. Don't think this is just a trick for fitness novices. It's good to use at any stage of a training journey to help feed and fuel your drive.

At the end of your workout, ask yourself:

8 QUESTIONS

1. Has my energy level increased?
2. Are there any places in my body that feel more comfortable now than when I started?
3. Has my breathing changed? (Am I taking fuller breaths or is it more rhythmic or relaxed?)
4. Has my mood changed? (Am I feeling any lighter, more hopeful, or more at ease?)
5. Has my level of anxiety or stress changed?
6. Does it feel easier to focus on what I'm

doing?

7. Do I feel better able to tackle the rest of the day ahead?

8. Do I have a greater sense of well-being?

I love the 8 questions because they bring you back to the very essence of why to work out in the first place: to feel better every day. As you proceed on your path, of course there will be other ways to track results. If you get on a focused training program such as the one I'll outline in chapter 6, you might experience changes in body composition, such as having less body fat and more muscle. Your clothes might fit differently, the circumferences of your torso and limbs may change, and your weight will likely change, too. You might find that your times and speeds on workouts improve, as do your personal bests of reps or weight.

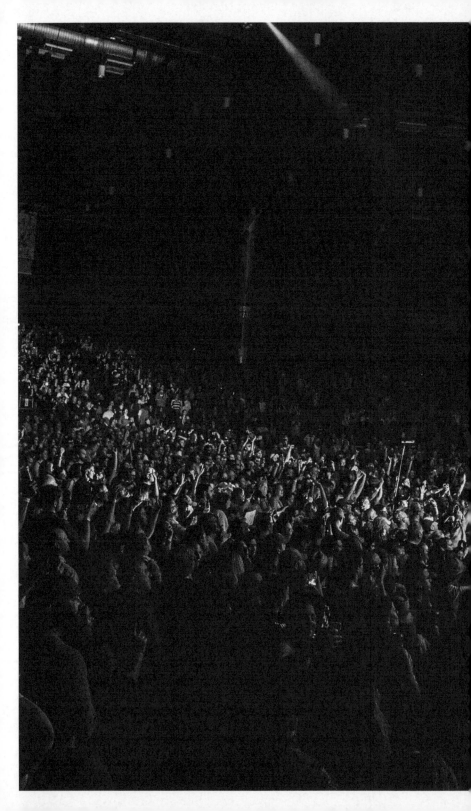

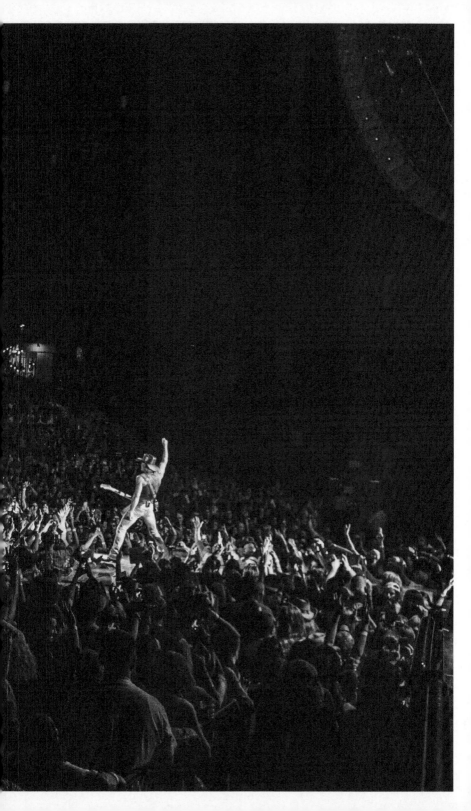

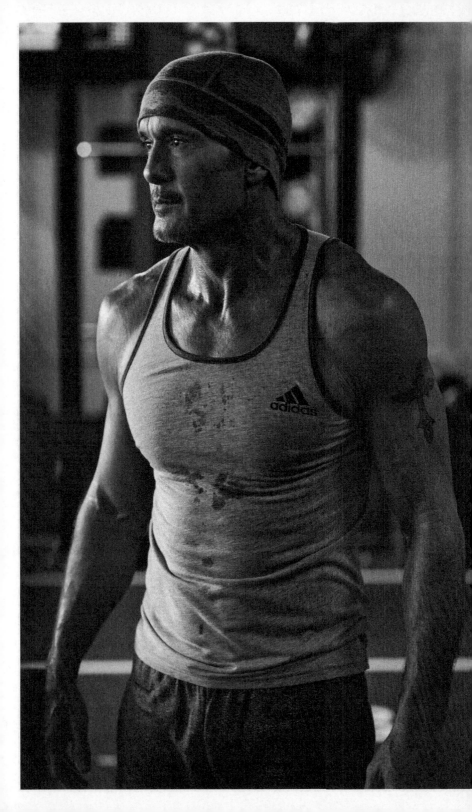

CHAPTER 4
DISCIPLINE

The ancient Chinese philosopher Lao Tzu said that the most important step on a thousand-mile journey is the first. I agree — to a point. If you *only* take the first step, you're not going to get very far. We all know that our impulsive brain can come up with a hundred and one reasons for quitting. So, if you want to be successful on your fitness journey, you have to plan a little further out than step one.

In my experience, the only way to do this is by building an infrastructure that guides the journey — I'm talking solid lanes and pathways that keep you on track throughout the process, with barrier walls installed so you don't bail out. This framework is made of the habits you cultivate. It's the nuts-and-bolts stuff: the advance preparation that helps you channel your intention into action, the planning that leaves as little as possible to chance.

If you're like me, you might initially balk at this idea. Committing to a fixed routine, creating a tight schedule, establishing habits — for some of us, those things feel alien. (If you're someone who loves a routine, then congratulations: You're naturally a systems person and you're going to feel right at home in this section of the book!) What I quickly learned as I committed to a fitness regimen is that when things get uncomfortable (as they inevitably will), you can't rely on willpower alone to make it through. You have to have a practical foundation in place that supports your goals. And maintaining that foundation requires discipline.

I rely on the predictability and structure of a routine to keep me grounded and tethered — and I'm gaining more and more respect for it with every trip around the sun. Life feels like it's speeding up for everyone, and that's doubly true when you're a musician on tour. When your whole environment changes from one day to the next — go to bed in one state, wake up in your tour bus in another — and when each stop involves a new city, a new arena, new press, new people, I can spin out quick. Having my same-old, time-tested routines solidly in place and following them with conviction is more than basic healthcare; it's my fast-acting remedy for when I get unsettled or unmoored. When too much is coming at me and I start to lose focus, I lean hard on my reliable routines of getting up early, working out, and eating in a way that fuels my performance. That is the basic support structure that carries me to the other side of any confusion or upset, letting me put my head down, do my work, and ride out the storm until I see clearly again. My routine serves another function that's invisible but essential: it acts as a lightning rod, attracting drive with all its motivating charge. Like a stake in the ground saying, *"Over here!,"* a consistent habit tells your drive when and where to show up to invigorate and inspire.

EMBRACING ROUTINE

When I began to create a fitness routine for myself, learning how to use discipline and routine to my advantage was my steepest learning curve. As with most hard lessons, though, it's one that's paid dividends over time. Discipline in fitness has led to a tidal wave of change rushing throughout my life. It tightened up my entire way of being, helping me be more productive and on point. I went from slightly sloppy — doing things how I felt like doing them, sometimes dropping the ball and often requiring others to wait or change plans — to a having more integrity all around.

Here's the thing: If you are going to own your health, you've got to have the foresight and the patience to fix all the leaks in the house. That includes the places where you give away your reserves by constantly negotiating with yourself about what to do. It also includes the harder-to-face leaks — the places where you lose the trust and willingness of others because you've failed to get all your bases covered and they end up having to accommodate your lateness, or your forgetting your word, or whatever other slipup has occurred from letting too many possibilities and ideas whirl around. Discipline truly is like a wrench set in my hand. I ask, "Where have I been getting a little too loose and sloppy?" Then, clamp, twist.

That said, I was a reluctant recruit to discipline and structure. I think that can partly be attributed to my childhood — growing up, those were two qualities pretty much absent from my life. My mom worked hard to provide for us kids and she did an incredible job, but frankly we were in survival mode for much of it, just getting by. Plus, it was a different time; we were on our own more than kids are today. Now that I'm a parent, I see clearly how kids thrive on structure and

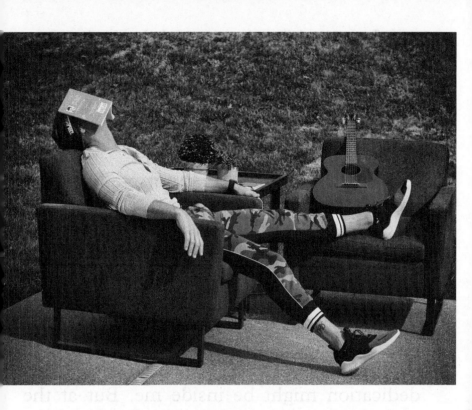

dedication might be inside me. But at the style of late nights and no

routine. I just didn't know what I was missing at the time.

Playing sports gave me the first taste of what structure felt like and, thank God, it gave me the framework I needed to do pretty well in school. Sports, I found, was all about systems: some outside authority figure creates the structure, and your job is to practice hard daily and show up without question for your coach and your team. But I had no clue how to implement those same types of systems after I graduated high school and was out on my own. Furthermore, I started hearing my second great passion calling to me: I wanted to play music! And who ever heard of a rock star laying out their clean jersey before bed and doing practice drills at dawn?

Looking back, I think it was that tension between the two sides of me — the athlete and the artist — that put me in a spin around discipline. The sports player in me revered the idea of physical sacrifice, order, and routine: By then I knew all about my dad, Tug, and the intensity he took to his training as a pitcher for the Mets and then the Phillies, helping both teams win the World Series. I had enough of an inkling about genes to know that some part of that dedication might be inside me. But at the same time, the artist in me wanted a lifestyle of late nights and no limits. I wanted to be free and without obligations, able to drop out of sight whenever the need to create might strike. The tension came to a head one day in my early twenties. I'd left college and was yo-yoing between two choices: Get legit and join the service, stepping into adulthood as a full-fledged marine recruit; or head to Nashville (which I knew virtually nothing about) and dive fearlessly into my bigger personal dream. I went down to my local recruitment office and filled out all the paperwork required to enlist, then went to bed that night feeling conflicted about what to do. The next morning, I woke up, grabbed my guitar, packed my bags, and bought a bus ticket. I arrived in Nashville the same night my country music hero, Keith Whitley, died and I never looked back.

That choice led me to something closer to rock-star life, where nobody but me could decide what I needed to do. Living on a schedule, waking up early, shutting down jam sessions to get to bed? No thanks. I loved being in the moment, putting everything I had into music. I liked the idea of being an "outlaw" or a "renegade." I don't regret it; losing discipline gave me the gift of figuring out how to find it, something I can now share with others. Plus, when you're young, you've got more expendable reserves. You can use them up and burn the candle at both ends to a degree. But getting older and merging my life with others — first Faith, then our three girls — meant maturing. Once things started getting messy, it became crystal clear that I had to get past my hang-ups and stop seeing structure and discipline as the enemy of creativity and the killer of passion.

When I turned things around, the athlete part of me spoke common sense to the artist, like a Little League coach talking to a kid with attitude. It said, "You *think* that putting routine and structure into your life will cramp your style, but you're wrong. You're kicking off a process of improving yourself, of making something great of your potential, of literally changing the tissues of your body and the way your cells use energy. You're changing the way your brain responds to the world and, in turn, your outlook on life. You're learning new skills and new ways of moving your body through space." This is a deep process and it requires practice. The definition of *practice* is something you do regularly, habitually, and whether it feels exciting or not. And to do it means taking all emotion out of the endeavor.

And anyway, I wasn't a kid at that point. I was in my mid-thirties and I had enough humility to know that my shoot-from-the-hip attitude was not as cute as it might have been when I was young and chasing my dream. Being sloppy as a family man and the leader of a music enterprise was irresponsible and self-centered. The renegade creates a cost that other people have to pay by adapting what they've planned or organized around you. That doesn't sit well with most.

I had to change my attitude, and my pledge to exercise daily for six weeks, every morning, no questions asked, was my hat-in-the-ring moment. As I turned my first six weeks into the next six then the next, I realized that I'd had it wrong. Discipline isn't punishing, and it's not about losing your edge. In fact, it doesn't require you to lose anything at all — it actually helps you gain the things you want the most. It's doesn't kill your dreams, it enables them. The Latin root of the word *discipline* means *"educate,"* and the education that you give yourself through discipline is the ability to overcome impulses to procrastinate, avoid, and quit. The ability to surrender the easy thing for the thing you actually want.

What I discovered was that discipline isn't something that certain people have, superachievers like my dad or Navy SEALS. Sure, some people embrace and thrive on structure and order more than others, and are more oriented to control. But discipline isn't a *trait* — it's a *skill set* that you develop through practice that gives you self-control and more authority over yourself, which in turn primes you to express more of yourself freely, not less. If I'm honest, I think I was always seeking discipline; I just didn't know how to get it.

DECISION FATIGUE

If you only subscribe to the idea of practicing the skills of discipline for one reason, let it be this: It spares you decision fatigue and helps you stop wasting your time. Trying to consistently make the right choice, the healthy choice, can feel like having a devil on one shoulder and an angel on the other. Until something's habitual and, better yet, nonnegotiable, your devil and your angel can get all riled up, going back and forth about the merits and justifications for ordering the lasagna over the grilled chicken, or binge-watching your favorite show versus getting out the dumbbells. It's exhausting to keep advocating for choices that, plain and simple, are going to help you live longer with more quality of life.

In music and art, that tension makes for good songs. Country music is full of stories of missteps, thrown-away chances, bad decisions, and redemption — they're timeless themes! In everyday life, however, the push-pull becomes draining. There's only so much mental energy you can put toward navigating the basics of a day before you get tapped out. That's a big reason we get stuck or fail to keep up healthy habits — we get burned out from battling about them inside. Either you're over it by day ten or you go hard at first, then give up, then start again, and that's not sustainable. Have you ever noticed how much of the energy you use for exercise drips into the most basic part: deciding whether or how to do it? When you insert structure and discipline where it was lacking, you short-circuit some of that old pattern. You create a routine that is nonnegotiable, so there's nothing to agonize over. That, to me, is the essence of discipline — it's actually something that makes your life easier, not harder.

And what a relief it is. Now you can put all that saved energy toward learning how to move, taking new classes, and discovering the best ways to work out for your body. The process becomes more fulfilling, which helps you keep at the new habit long enough to get past the initial bumps and find your groove. And when you're also acknowledging any boosts in how you feel — using the 8 questions on page 170–171, for example — repeating the ritual really starts to pay back. It rewires your brain, which begins to create reward chemistry in *anticipation* of doing the exercise, because it's learned how good it's going to feel. That's how you get a positive snowball effect. What was once a chore becomes a habit that feels good enough to continue and, over time, a passion you don't want to live without.

My initial six-week challenge helped the fog clear from my eyes. I liked feeling successful in a small way every day. And I sure liked feeling physically better and happier in my body every day. That was enough to motivate me to lay down a structure that doesn't change much. At home, mornings are my time to work out, whether I have forty-five minutes, an hour, or some days the luxury of even longer workouts — a special bonus of my career, which I don't take for granted. I head into them the same way each time, layering up first because I like to sweat — sweatpants, long-sleeve T-shirt, and sweatshirt, unless it's already hot and humid out. I start with walking to loosen up, shake off sleep, and help my body remember its rhythm, then do my mobility warm-up and then my workout. On the road this routine becomes multipart, because now I'm in peak performance mode. The walk in the morning is followed by a forty-five-minute workout on the stadium stairs before lunch with Roger if he's traveling with us, then the hour-plus group workout in the afternoon — our energy-raising, camaraderie-boosting team training ritual.

The key is that every day's fitness and health choices are pretty well mapped out and everyone knows the drill — it doesn't change unless something truly unexpected occurs. The workouts are no longer the

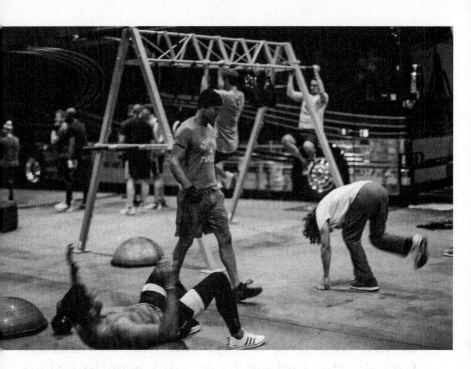

afterthought; they're the starting block from which the rest of the day unfolds. And luckily, the people around me help make that reality happen because, if you quiz them, they'll probably tell you, organizing the health and fitness chunks of my day have made me a much more organized person in general. It's helped my brain to like knowing what's happening in advance and have chunks of the day separated and timed almost to the minute. I get a lot more done in a month than I used to, even with the added time devoted to exercise. Now I'm the one with the eye on the clock, starting the conference call on the minute, shaving off seconds where I can.

I should note here that my version of self-control doesn't resemble living like a hard-core Marine or an austere monk, giving up life's comforts. For a routine to stick, it has to feel good. In the end, it's just about making the best choices you can that will help you build the life you want, instead of falling into behaviors that pull you further away from that goal. Discipline doesn't have to mean conformity or rigidity. For me it's opened up more free space, more potential for creativity and flow.

Honestly, I don't think I'm the exception to the rule. I've always felt that the harder I work, the luckier I get, and creating clear frameworks for getting the hard work done has helped everything exponentially improve. Funny, I've come to see how the best creativity is a "same time, same place" kind of phenomenon. It's less about getting lost in feeling, and more about showing up daily to write or practice at the piano. The same idea applies if your art is your life; the great moments come because you show up the same way for your family, your friends, or your business reliably, calmly, predictably. The magic isn't sourced in living like you're wildly inspired all the time or on a high-low roller coaster of drama! It happens when you put in the time on the jobs that need to get done and stay in the grind long enough so that, for brief moments, the magic happens: The melody comes into your mind that perfectly expresses what's in your heart; the sweet connection happens between you and your kids; the solution to a problem drops into your mind.

When you have the discipline to stick with the effort consistently, you set up the conditions and open the door for inspiration to find *you*. And that's what helps you perform in a way that transcends the ordinary, whether it's in art, at work, as a parent, or as a friend. Maturity is accepting that you do the hard work most of the time to have the peak moments some of the time. And you know what? Being more conventional in my day-to-day lifestyle in this way has made for a healthier kind of artistry. I've gained more objective distance, more space, and more clarity. If I want to sing about heartbreak and suffering, I can sing about it, but I don't have to live in it.

I've come to develop an appreciation for humble old discipline, but I don't take it for granted. I watch it and myself like a hawk. Because here's the thing about discipline: you gotta keep working at it, keep taking care of your routines and your dedication to them, because as soon as you quit thinking about them or think you have it all nailed, routine and commitment will try to slip away. Staying disciplined is a work in progress that doesn't stop. And while that obviously involves *work,* it's also what keeps pouring benefits into the rest of your life.

THE 7 PILLARS OF DISCIPLINE

All structures need pillars for support and stability. When it comes to building a workout routine, you need to put several pillars in place, so that if one gets wobbly or stressed, the others still hold you. Think of them as implementing daily rituals to your life. Rituals not only add order and structure to your hectic days but also inspire your mind to stay focused on your priorities and your heart to keep calling in your drive. I've got seven of them.

1. Microgoals

Travels tend to go easier when there are places to stop at — benches where you take a breath, check in with how it's going, and then plot the next segment of the trip. Setting microgoals helps break down the bigger dream of wanting to be fit and strong into actionable chunks. It's easier to stay on the path when you aim for destinations that are well within sight; it also gives you moments of satisfaction and happiness frequently, which function as positive feedback to help you stay engaged. If you've ever played golf and gone to a driving range, you know how good it feels to hit a hundred balls and see your swing improve. Microgoals are like that — they give you small-scale satisfactions to balance out the patience and frustrations involved with mastering the full-length game. They also help prevent against the trap of going too fast too soon; going slower and steadier out of the gate helps you make it to a reasonable checkpoint instead of speeding recklessly towards your ideal body and new life, throwing everything you have at the dream but risking injury, burnout, and loss of interest or heart as a result.

My first microgoal was to complete six weeks of morning walks, but even within that I broke it down into weekly microgoals. Do seven days; now do another. When that was complete and I felt the trust in my abilities return, I set the next one: Do one month of ramping up to circuit training by improving my form and technique on all the basic moves I'd need as well as mastering new movements like kettlebell swings. And the microgoal setting went on from there: Do three circuit training sessions a week plus two long walks, for three weeks; then add in strength training sessions at strategic intervals. Sometimes the microgoal was performance based: complete one of my favorite circuits 20 percent faster this month or increase the weight I'm using by a certain number of pounds.

Now that working out is second nature, I still set microgoals all the time — the requirements of my job make it happen. If a tour is coming up, I look at the calendar, evaluate my current fitness level and how close I am to my fighting strength and weight, and create a series of goals to guide me to my best tour shape. If a video shoot is coming up, I pull back my lens and look at my eating habits, and make a dietary microgoal to throw cheat foods out the window for two weeks. If I want to develop strength in particular part of my body, like my back, my core, or my legs, I have the know-how to add in extra focus there. And other times it's just to learn using a new piece of equipment and to get really good at it.

A microgoal strategy will help you more effectively than making one gigantic but amorphous goal to change your life, stat! There's too much pressure and not enough specificity in those types of resolutions. The trick is to take a breath and trust that incremental steps, even if they seem small, truly add up over time. A key aspect of microgoals is that they help you progress — so it's smart to think about the big picture and plot out how you'll get there. In chapter 6, I'll give you a template for workouts that gradually build your endurance and strength. But no matter what type of exercise or practice you're doing, you can look at it with this perspective. What do you want to achieve? Break off a small piece of that big goal, chew it well, savor it, get the nutrition out of it, then break off the next piece. Here are two things to keep in mind.

If you're new to fitness: Be realistic, and be gentle with yourself. It's okay to start small when you're aiming to establish the habit. Tame the part of you that thinks you have to GO BIG OR GO HOME right out the gate. Even top trainers agree that clients are more successful when they downgrade expectations and start by making the habit as easy as possible to achieve. At first that may mean ten to fifteen minutes of daily movement, like walking or doing the mobility drills on pages 318–341. Maybe it's literally doing fifteen minutes of breathing, moving, and gentle walking at home or at your gym, three times a week. That doesn't mean you have to stop at fifteen minutes if you're feeling great, but anything after fifteen minutes is gravy. You met your microgoal and it's okay to stop. This is a powerful strategy because it gives you a small easy victory, avoids stress and anxiety, and builds your confidence that you can do what you set out to do. Roger likes to break the lifestyle down into 21-day chunks: Commit to a 21-day cycle of one kind of activity (walking, swimming, body-weight strength training); achieve it, then commit to the next 21-day cycle. It looks good on a wall calendar and is long enough to become a new normal, but short enough to feel achievable. Cycle by cycle, you link together a whole new lifestyle.

If you're active and want to optimize your habit: Set microgoals that are achievable, but not so easy to achieve that you can go on cruise control. They need to challenge you because challenge is where growth occurs — physically and mentally — and it's also what keeps the mind engaged and excited. It might be to do an online workout four times a week; or to work with a coach on strength-training skills that seem out of reach. The point is to find a sweet spot where your goals test you but don't crush you. Sometimes it's helpful to get some guidance from a professional or from a community of workout enthusiasts (see page 222). There's nothing wrong with looking to others who are further along than you and using their feats to set your own benchmarks. Just make sure you have a strategy for progressing there safely and effectively.

Whatever level you're at, remember the power of the pen. Writing down your goals makes them several steps closer to being

SMALL GOALS, MAJOR PROGRESS

Try sprinkling micromovement goals throughout your day. This not only supports your health from multiple angles but also helps you get a taste for setting goals and meeting them. A microgoal might be to have a day of constantly returning to good posture at your desk, to set a timer to remind you to take a minute of full, deep breaths every twenty minutes, to get up and move every forty-five minutes, or to drink eight glasses of water a day. If you want to take it up a level and build strength, set a microgoal of doing five perfect-form push-ups every time you go to the kitchen or bathroom. Succeeding at these micro-goals helps you see that you can "do discipline" and gives your upward cycle of health a boost. It's about small movement victories, done through conscious choice.

manifest; at the very least, it keeps them at the front of your mind.

2. Consistency

I met Johnny Paycheck years ago when I was starting out in the business. Paycheck was one of the true outlaws of country music's Outlaw movement. His most well-known hit, "Take This Job and Shove It," gives you a little hint at the fire in his personality. We were all hanging out on the front of my bus and I was eager to get any advice he'd give me about how to successfully navigate a long career. He told me, "Son, just make sure you get up enough speed so that when you hit the ditch, you come out the other side." We all laughed that night, but I knew just what he meant. There'd be uptimes and downtimes ahead, but if I could get enough momentum, I could plow through the bumps and keep moving forward.

I feel the same way about working out. Get momentum going at all costs up front so that the bumps in the road that come — inevitably and frequently — don't throw you for a loop. Real life is unpredictable, things come up, people need us in a different way today from yesterday. Getting momentum makes you more resilient to those surprises, and the way you get it is by committing to consistency: Deciding to do your chosen practice regularly — ideally, some kind of movement daily, and definitely not letting more than a day or two go by between sessions. Consistency is actually *more* important than intensity or complexity: It's better to do something simple regularly than to do an epic push once a every few months. (As you get more advanced, consistently tapping intensity and complexity will be part of your program.)

It doesn't take a master's degree to figure out consistency, but it does take pointed effort. Schedule your exercise into your week, blocking out the time in advance. If it's possible to use the same time slots repeatedly — or even the same time every day — it will help you find your rhythm more easily. This doesn't mean that *what* you do necessarily has to be the same — it could alternate between walking, yoga, and circuit training — but having the time block carved for it tells your body and mind it's coming. I know it might sound a little crazy, but I feel my whole self getting ready for this standing date like a dog knowing its walk is coming. My mind starts to turn away from the news of the day and toward the workout, and I could swear my heart rate increases a bit and my breath deepens in advance. Routine helps me feel ready.

Personally, I prefer morning workouts. Though it can feel tough to get started, I find that moving my body in the morning sets me up for success. I can go about the rest of my day knowing I've gotten the hardest part done — physically, at least — and I feel lighter and sharper all day long. If I left my workout until later, there'd be a lot more opportunities for intrusions and unexpected events to change the plan. Plus, with so much else going on, I'd have to work harder to focus and get my energy devoted to working out. I've learned how morning exercise helps your body dial down cortisol levels and keep them at a lower level all day; maybe that's why my stress management is better when I work out first thing versus later in the day.

But find what works for you — and your kids and dogs, your carpools and commutes. Experiment with different schedules and see what you can achieve with the least angst and most efficiency — predawn; lunch hour; baby's nap time; after school at the playground; while dinner cooks and the kids do homework. The workouts in the next section can be done in as little as twenty minutes. The only caution: Don't leave your fitness session until too late in the day, because working out vigorously within a couple of hours of bedtime can mean you'll have a harder time falling asleep.

Nothing's more awkward than fumbling to find a rhythm — in music or in life. Teach the instrument of your body to expect a regular beat, beat, beat, and before you know it, it (and you) will come to look forward to it.

3. Communication

Part of achieving consistency and building momentum is telling others what you need. That can feel uncomfortable, especially if you've got a lot of demands and expectations on your plate or are used to always being there for your family, friends, and colleagues. But clear your throat and speak up. This is about claiming time and space to take care of yourself first — and rest assured, it's an oxygen-mask scenario. When you make your own health a top priority, you're a lot more capable at tending to the health and well-being of others.

What you're seeking is support and respect: other people don't have to want the same thing for themselves or even understand your choices, but you do need them to honor your personal process of building your best state of health. Half an hour, forty minutes, an hour some days — even if it's broken into segments — this is how you're investing in being the most stable, calm, and clear-headed version of yourself you can be. Those around you will reap the rewards.

It's tough at first. But to win that support, you might have to explain why this matters. Get clear on the "whys" that you feel comfortable sharing — chances are, they'll be the rational reasons more than the passion — and practice articulating them so you can own your needs confidently. If you feel yourself choking on your words, it's worth asking where that limitation comes from: Who ever said you don't deserve the time to protect and improve your health? Maybe even more important, share the results you're getting. Your loved ones may be able to sense the changes in your mood, energy, focus, or clarity. They may even see the results in your skin, your eyes, and eventually your waistline. Or they may not. Don't expect anyone to be a mind reader. Tell them how much better you're feeling from getting regular exercise, share what's going right. When others find out how it's helping you, they're much more likely to have your back.

My family and I have our share of tussles when my daily workout causes a hitch in our morning plans. Fortunately, they like fit Tim much better than frustrated Tim, so we generally work things out, with a laugh or two. The bigger issue for me in this process for me was learning to say no to the stuff that seemed important, and maybe was important — but wasn't more important than my health. Prioritizing business and professional demands, turning down opportunities, letting the leader in me draw boundaries, trusting that enough was enough. To own your health, I discovered, you have to get fearless about drawing a line. Of course, if you're a busy parent or caregiver, or if you're juggling work, studies, and commutes, even drawing a line can feel like a luxury. Nobody's handing you a pen. In those cases you have to do some slash-and-burn on any pockets of minutes that get used up on lower priorities. If you feel like you don't have enough time to walk or work out, consider doing an audit of your free time. Where do you fritter away minutes on social media or watching a show that doesn't get you anywhere? Five minutes there, three minutes here, and seven minutes there get close to adding up to a short workout.

More ruthlessly, where do you give your time and energy away to people or things who aren't close to your core or deeply held part of your values — maybe just because you're being nice, or trying to be polite? There's no easy way around it: you might have to take an ax to the forest and let a little light in. Sometimes it involves speaking frankly to your kids: You love them and value their needs and wants, but they need to value yours. If that means giving up something they'd like to do so you can work out, maybe that's a lesson well learned. You're modeling something healthy to them by taking care of your well-being for the long haul. Other times, it means clearing your throat and asking for help. That friend who offered to babysit, or your sister who owes you one? Cash in those chips and set up a system. Maybe they'd even like to participate in a fitness plan, swapping days of childcare so each one of you can exercise. If everyone seems too caught up in their problems to help, or too busy to accommodate you, you're probably part right. But it's up to you to cut through the distraction and get their attention, and then hear their needs, too. Remember the higher goal here is health, happiness, and having more to give — what if we all talked about it directly and helped each other get there?

4. Plans

Among the many Sharpie scribbles on my home gym mirrors are lists of movements — overhead press x 5, loaded front squat x

7 — that I've organized into the workout of the day. If I'm on the road, we mimic this with a whiteboard or sometimes a scrap of paper. But the point is, there's a plan for the action that's been thought through.

Planning a workout for the day is something I learned from high school athletics; Coach Butler always had our training sequences mapped out before we hit the field. When I took charge of my own fitness all those years later, it felt a little clumsy at first, because I was still new to understanding how to make a well-rounded drill that

PREP FOR SUCCESS

One of the best ways to make your workout plan rock solid is to prep everything you need in advance, ideally the night before. Get your clothes, shoes, water bottle, and anything else ready to go, and place them by your bedroom door or the front door. If you change and shower at the gym, make sure to pack a bag with your gear and any other essentials so you don't leave anything to chance in the morning, when things can get hectic. The more prepared you are, the less likely you will be to make excuses or bail.

checked the right boxes for the day. But I got better at it over time, and now choreographing the morning's workout is one of my favorite parts of the process. I do it the night before so that when daylight comes it's nailed down: there's no dancing around, losing time, staring at stuff in the gym. I plot out how I want to warm up, what my workout will be, how I'll transition between exercises, and how long I'll rest in between. I even think about how I want to cool down after. There's an arc sketched out so that I can drop in and go.

Deciding what you're going to do the next day is pivotal to maintaining momentum. First, it makes you a lot more likely to show up for it — studies show that explicitly stating what you're going to do, when you'll do it, and where and how you'll do it helps to boost self-regulation and control. Once you start, it keeps you moving.

This approach isn't for experts only. It's worth doing even if your goal is to walk the next day or you'll only have a few minutes for some squats, planks, and shoulder rolls as you get ready for work. Imagine what time you'll do these things, where, and for how long. If you like doing classes, plan them out and register in advance if necessary. And if the idea of choreographing a high-intensity

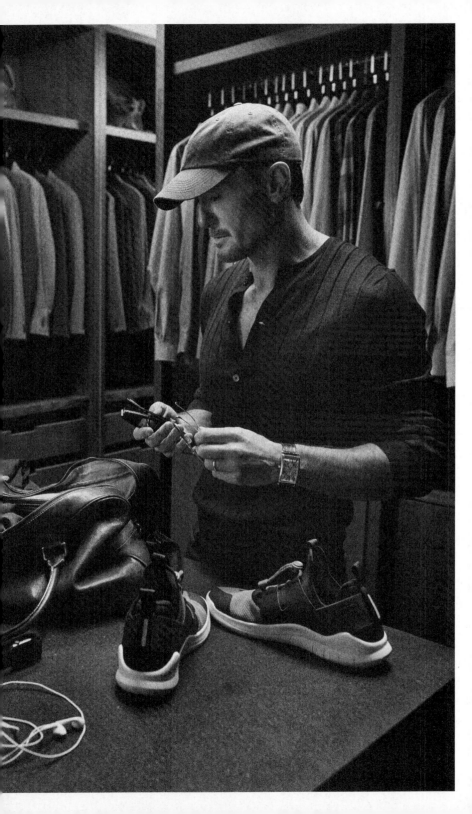

or strength-building workout seems out of reach, maybe your plan is to do a workout from this book or to stream a workout from one of the many fitness sites online. Even planning seven minutes of mobility warm-ups while your kid gets dressed for school and before walking to the bus can be surprisingly effective. It makes small routines of well-being into rituals you anticipate.

Planning your workouts in advance — as opposed to getting up early to "work out," unsure if you're heading out for a run or going to the gym — keeps your good intentions and plans on track. Icy roads or hazardous windstorms predicted? You know about it because you checked the weather the day before — and, naturally, you made a plan to skip your outdoor run and work out in your basement. Having a tiring week of travel or hard deadlines? A high-voltage kickboxing class may feel too overwhelming, better to schedule a yoga class you'll look forward to instead. Had a lonely few days? Sign up to take a group class or meet a friend or two for a hike.

5. Accountability

I have a good friend named Mark who lives across the country from me. We have a relationship that is deep and meaningful even though it's carried out through extremely short, to-the-point text messages. It goes something like this:

Tim: Bar Complex today.
Mark (60 minutes later): Done.
Tim: Fist-pump emoji.

Mark and I fell into this buddy system after I hooked him into the workout habit some years ago, and now we keep each other accountable. I know he's waiting for my daily text with a special challenge for our workouts, and I feel too much responsibility to let him down, and vice versa — once he sees my message, he's got too much pride to let it go unreturned. This keeping our eyes on each other, digitally at least, works in our both our favors; it's a support system for helping each of us meet our goals.

Accountability is the glue that keeps you on your healthy path. There's a whiff of obligation to it: you've entered some kind of agreement to report yourself, to answer to someone or something about your actions. Some people are wholly accountable to themselves and don't need to answer to anyone — their motivation to succeed just dominates and they'd never miss a workout. But if that's not you — and frankly, it's not most people — having another human witness your microgoal and then hold you accountable to it is really helpful.

Building in accountability can be as simple as voicing your exercise plan to your partner or friend. Even saying aloud what you intend to do is useful; it puts you on the spot if you come up short, and who wants that? Once you put words to something, you feel like you're cheating yourself if you don't do it. If you and your partner or friend work out together, this gets even stronger — you both sign up, and now you don't want to let the other down.

But sometimes you have to step it up a notch and put more on the line than words. Here are a few ways to get a little more skin in the game.

1 FINANCIAL ACCOUNTABILITY:
Backing up your goal with cash is a great incentive to stay committed. But since a lot of people join a gym and then don't go, sometimes dues alone aren't enough. One option to up the ante: Pay for a coach or series of nonrefundable classes in advance (a coach is ideal, because they'll also give you a hard time if you don't show). Alternatively, go maverick: place a bet with a friend on who will

be the first to miss a mutually planned workout — loser hands over the cash — or you can even do the now-legendary "negative charity" trick. Pledge a painful amount of money to a cause you detest, should you fail to meet your microgoal. That'll keep you on the straight and narrow.

2 SOCIAL ACCOUNTABILITY: Sign up for a charity event that requires training, and get supporters on board to sponsor your cause — you won't want to disappoint them. Make a public pledge on your social media about your current goal, and ask friends to follow along (and support you) as you update with milestones. Be open about the ups and downs — it solicits more engagement. Ask a fellow team member to keep tabs on you; see if they'll program your workout time into their calendar for two or three weeks and check up on you via text or e-mail until your habit's established.

3 PHYSICAL ACCOUNTABILITY: Find a way to track changes in your body composition through images or measurements. If you are comfortable with it, having photos of yourself in workout gear that you store in a folder on your computer or phone lends a serious kick in the butt — whether you're seeking to lose fat or add more mass. Alternatively, measure the circumference of your arms, legs, chest, waist, and hips and keep a tally of inches lost or gained, checking every two months or so for change. If you want to get really geeky, you can set a body fat percentage goal you hope to achieve — but checking this accurately requires professional help, such as measurement in a Bod Pod device. Using a scale to see what change is occurring can be deceptive because of the disparity that occurs when you first lose fat and put on muscle; the number might go up as you start putting on muscle, because muscle weighs more than fat even though it's more compact, taking up less space. The thing is, you need that extra muscle to help burn the fat — it's a metabolic driver. So it's smarter, at first, to ditch the scales and pay attention to how you feel and look. I've come to know my ideal set point in weight, and the numbers tell me if I've been slacking and gained a bit or if I'm overdoing it on the cardio and losing too much mass. The number on the scale gives me a quick clue about what's going on, though it's taken some self-study to get to this place. But by far the simplest way to track changes in body composition? Let the fit of your clothes be your guide, especially any changes in fit around the middle, which is where fat accumulates most easily when your metabolism is off balance. It's free, it's fast, and the fit doesn't lie. It doesn't hurt to have some clothes you want to wear when you've become a leaner, meaner fat-burning machine — or at least maybe that's what I tell myself to justify all the suits in my closet.

4 **TECHNOLOGY ACCOUNTABILITY:** FitBits, Apple watches, and other devices that measure your steps, output, pace; heart rate monitors used during a conditioning workout to show you how hard you're working; online circuit workouts that let you punch in the reps you did to be saved for later comparison — today there are multiple ways to monitor your achievements on a screen. There are lots of different apps for runners and cyclists that let you track and analyze your workouts using your phone or GPS watch, measure your performance, join challenges with others, share photos,

and follow friends. Old-schoolers use a low-tech paper and pencil and a clock on the wall to record their progress in speed or load. Either way, tracking how you're performing and seeing hard numbers can help you maintain the mojo to keep pursuing your goals.

5 REWARD ACCOUNTABILITY: Promise yourself a treat if you complete your microgoal. It's not just horses that chase carrots — we all step up the pace if a prize is in sight. It can be simple: your favorite green juice or great cup of coffee if you make it to morning spin class, or trying a new restaurant if you made it to after-work kettlebells. Or it can be a reward like a massage if you do boot camp three times a week, or a candlelight restorative yoga class. Ready to go all out? Write a bigger reward into your future, like a hiking or biking trip somewhere you've always wanted to go — or as I did with flying, learning something you've always wanted to master. The more varied the rewards, the better the reward center of your brain responds, causing the feel-good chemistry of anticipation and satisfaction to surge at the idea of exercising.

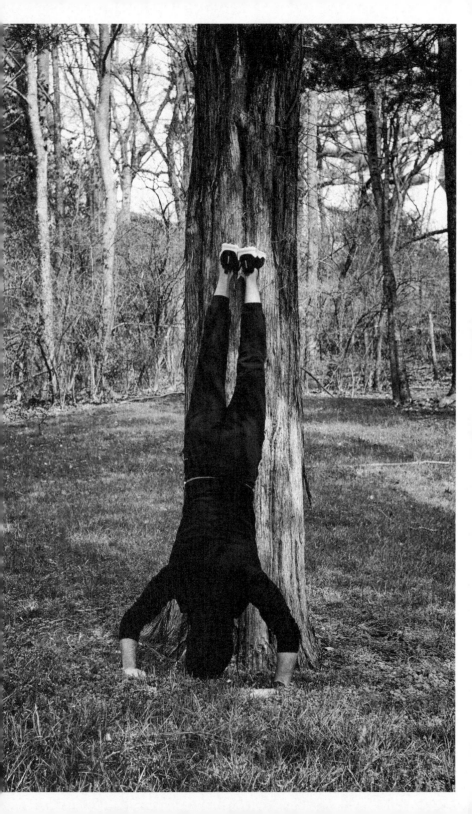

6. Creativity

A ladder bolted to the wall of a stadium; a set of monkey bars at the park; that massive bag of dog food you just purchased at the feed store. And yes, the bumper of an 18-wheeler truck. What do these things have in common? They're all examples of exercise equipment waiting to be commandeered for your workout, if you can just see them with fresh eyes.

The successful athlete is the improvisational athlete — someone who creates the conditions to move no matter the circumstances. When the massive black TRUMAV gym trailer isn't at his disposal, fiddle player Dean will get his box jumps going on the boulders at a nearby park and do pull-ups, dips, and hanging leg raises on nearby play structure — providing no small humans have claimed it as their own. The sandbags stashed in your garage? They're weights that cost nothing and work well for impromptu farmer carries, loaded front squats, and more. And the ladder and giant bumper — those were memorable parts of an upper-body sequence I choreographed during a workout in Austin.

Creativity feeds a successful practice because it ensures that you dodge two common pitfalls on the fitness path: skipping exercise because you "can't make it" to a legit facility or fancy gym; or losing momentum and hitting a plateau because you're getting bored. Make the environment around you into your gym! Rocks, trees, park benches, hills for sprinting — they're gifts for the flexible athlete. And the dog food? Sling it over your shoulder and do a series of 50-meter walks, with a few burpees in between. Those things and much more are available if you're a movement opportunist, keeping your eyes open for new ways to lift, carry, push, and pull.

Even if you reliably do have access to a nice, controlled place to work out, a creative attitude lets you mix things up when your desire is flagging. It's one of the rare times I think falling down an Instagram wormhole can be of service: The right feeds from a reputable trainer can show you new movements you never thought of, and help you mix up the angles and planes of movement you're working in. Switching up these variables can deliver big payback, as they make your body adapt to new kinds of stresses. And making something harder, if you're in the right shape for it, is a good way to overcome plateaus and increase motivation. I know I've hit it right if I'm sore in a whole new way the next day.

Creativity is also key for "play," an aspect of health that can get overlooked when you're mainly focused on getting your workouts in. Play, which we'll look at in chapter 6, is unstructured movement done purely for the joy of it. The kind of stuff that brings out your inner kid. So train yourself to see your environment through the eyes of a child. What can you to jump on, run under, or engage with? When you bring fresh perspective to your surroundings, there's no room for excuses.

7. Community

The last of the 7 pillars may just be the most important one. Sharing the journey with others keeps you firmly on your path. When even *one* other person shares the workout experience with you, something special happens: you raise each other's energy, and you cheerlead and coach each other to improve and progress.

It can be lonely when you turn toward a healthier, more active lifestyle; it's likely that not everyone in your world feels the same motivation that you do. So create your own network of people who have your back and want you to succeed and are actively living the lifestyle you want for yourself. Surround yourself with people — or even just one person at first — who feed your flame and aren't trying to snuff it out.

For my sister Sandy, community came through starting a walking group of women who meet after the daily school run in a park in Nashville on the days she's not doing circuit training at the gym. She calls the group her support system for staying healthy; she and her friends walk their way to mental clarity and energy. This group habit has so impacted the focus she brings to her workday, she attributes it to the professional success she's experienced since her own health turning point six years ago.

Community building is a huge part of the reason we have the TRUMAV trailer parked outside our tour venues, available to anyone on our tour staff who has the inclination to join us. It's a group-think thing, or maybe a gravitational pull. The communal workout amplifies the drive to work hard — as if everyone throws some of their individual drive in the pot and it compounds and grows in force — everyone feels the positive vibe and starts hopping around in anticipation of how fun-slash-hard-slash rewarding this is going to be. That's no small thing: If you're going to sprint, crawl, or Komodo push your way up the inclined grassy lawns where the audience will sit later, you need all the extra juice in your tank you can get. Doing this with friends who are fitter than you and adding a jolt of friendly competition gives an extra boost: research shows that people output up to 200 percent more effort when their workout partners set a high bar, which is important because to truly make gains in strength and fitness, you need to push beyond what was possible before. Plus, studies show that those who are overweight lose more weight when they spend time with fitter, healthier friends. Communal workouts, like creativity,

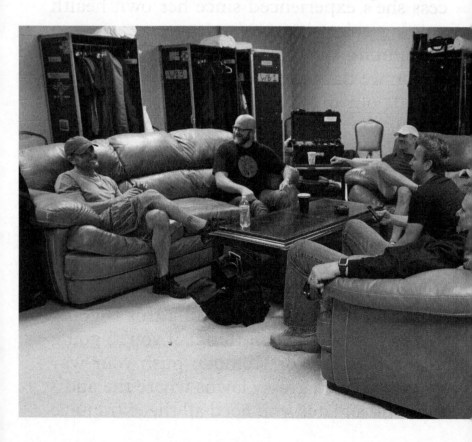

also help squelch the primary reason people quit their exercise habit: boredom. You're less likely to get into a rut when a group and/or a coach or teacher has a few hundred workout innovations up their sleeve.

Sweating together has bonded us in a way we'd never quite achieved when we simply knew each other casually from the music scene. Sometimes there are twenty people devoting themselves to a workout, motivating one another or keeping an eye on each other's form and technique. In between circuits as we let our heart rates stabilize, we talk about topics as free-ranging as our families, our pasts, and what happened in the show the night before. We laugh and rib each other, too, which adds to that cocktail of well-being chemistry produced during exercise — when you laugh, dopamine is released in the perfectly balanced amount to give you a "natural high," which is why laughing feels so good! Laughter combined with movement may just be the world's best medicine.

There's a unique kind of camaraderie and fellowship you generate when you're all in it together, stripped down to your tank tops. Differences in status or role are put to one side, and everyone's equally invested in the same cause: pushing himself or herself to achieve. A few hours later, when we start playing our show, my band mates and I are more connected and in sync, and — proof that structure frees you up to express yourself fully — we're more playful and spontaneous, too. Working our bodies together earlier in the day has opened another dimension to our musicality, and it can feel like magic — being totally in tune with what we're all about to do.

Another benefit of community fitness? It anchors accountability. Once the daily rhythm is established, nobody wants to be the weak link who bails on the rest, so consistency is easier to achieve. Especially for me! When I know a bunch of people are expecting a good workout at the appointed time, I don't waffle. After all, I'm the quarterback, and if the quarterback doesn't show up, nobody else will. I'm grateful for that peer pressure — bearing the torch for our daily workouts adds to my sense of purpose.

What my bandmates and I didn't expect when we started this was how contagious it would prove to be. It's not uncommon for our support acts to sniff around us for a minute, wondering what the heck we're up to. Next thing you know we've got them roped in. That exposure to our culture of healthy living inspired their own upward cycle. I'm pretty sure that's why Dean, Denny, Billy, and Paul say the group workouts have been life-changing; having a net of support has carried them further in their health goals than they could have gone on their own.

Community can look all kinds of ways, but to my mind, there's no substitute for gathering in the flesh. The obvious starting point: enlisting your family, partner, or best friends to consistently join your exercise mission. A regular class of your favorite type of exercise can help, too. Best of all is finding a fitness, sport, or movement family of some kind, one that has a culture of its own. That means a place where people congregate regularly not just to burn calories but also to develop themselves and master new skills, typically with all levels welcome and more experienced players mentoring the new ones in some way. A place where relationships are prized as much as physical results.

This might be a CrossFit box or running club, but it could also be a lunchtime workout group you create at your workplace, a new-parent boot camp in the park, or your local Hike it Baby chapter, which gets parents and caregivers outside on trails wearing their infants or walking their toddlers. It could be a yoga studio that encourages engagement through workshops or partnering up in classes. A Masters Swim training group, a triathlon training group, or a rock-climbing gym that leads you to start climbing outside on excursions over time can also forge bonds. A martial-arts dojo that mixes practitioners of different belts can put you in the position of learning from your peers,

ASK QUESTIONS

If you're new to exercise, it's important to ask a trainer, coach, or staff member at your gym or fitness studio about the right starting place for you. If you're interested in taking a class, ask for help in matching the activity with your skill level (and when in doubt, it's a good idea to default to cardio classes, which are generally safer for beginners than strength training classes, where attention to form is paramount to prevent injuries). Don't be shy about asking for extra help and being direct with trainers to ensure you are doing any exercises properly and safely. And if the people you're dealing with can't answer your questions or don't make you feel comfortable, look for another place to train where you can benefit from the support and guidance of experienced professionals.

then teaching them yourself. And if none of these things are possible, do what Sandy did: Start something yourself; get the word out through friends, social media, or your kids' school; then see who comes.

It can be intimidating to go from solo to group if you feel you're not the joining kind or you're worried you don't have the experience to put yourself out there in public. Push past that fear: The right group will embrace you and get you ramped up safely and slowly. Moving together isn't just about meeting fitness goals, it's about benefiting from the qualities of group fitness that might be the most health-giving of all: connection and belonging.

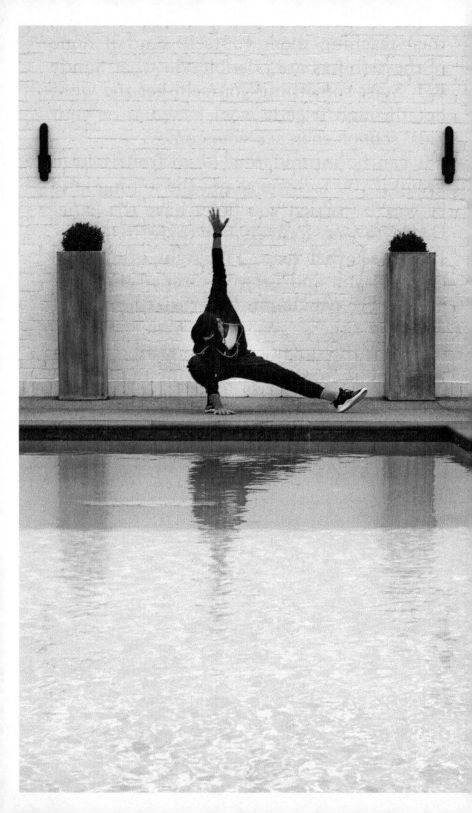

CHAPTER 5
DEEP FOCUS

Back when I was a high school athlete, I started a curious habit. I'd lie in my bed at night visualizing every detail of the next day's practice or game. If it was baseball, I'd go through each possible scenario of how to turn my body so I'd make every catch; how to change my foot position so I'd be at the perfect angle for every throw from shortstop to first, second, or third. If it was basketball, I'd imagine sinking the winning basket, seeing the ball leaving my hands and swishing clean through the net over and over, the entire play unfolding in slow motion. Playing it all out in my head in advance and visualizing every piece of the game helped me feel as prepared as I could be. Then, in the heat of the moment, all that focus and preparation let me tap into a state of flow. Once the game started, I could stop trying and thinking so hard and hand over the reins to my senses, my reflexes, and my muscles.

When I started performing live music, I didn't have anyone coaching me on how to do a good show. So I migrated that habit over from field to stage. I started doing advance run-throughs, imagining in detail what it'd feel like when the lights blaze on and where the band would be and how I'd move to where I needed to go. To this day, I use this ritual to prepare for a great show. Each song plays out in my mind, and I can see the moment my head will turn this way or my hand will gesture that way. I'll focus in on the particular mood I want to express through my gait or the way a certain phrase gets intoned. Maybe it will suddenly hit me how the lighting needs to change to make the audience feel more reflective or how the outro of the song has to be longer, so the last line lingers and makes you think. I want to get the most impact from the smallest things and tell a story with a few simple gestures.

When it gets close to showtime, I put on my black hat as carefully as I used to put on my team jersey. That hat is a cue that tells my mind, *Game on.* All doubts or hesitations about myself as an artist or a dad or a husband get put on hold. There's a big match to win and I've got to give it everything I've got. Even up to the last moment before the show, pacing the backstage hallways to shake

226

off any nerves, I'm picturing getting onstage with my friends, watching the crowd light up, and I imagine all of us feeling that physical surge that shoots through you when you know you're going to have a blast.

Visualization is what helps me focus my mind and connect deeply to my body so that I stop overthinking and drop into a state of flow. It mentally prepares me so that the best performance I have to give can find its way out. Coach Butler used to say, "Make practice harder than the game, so when game time comes, you can play natural and easy." Taking the time to get my mind locked in is as much of a part of that practice as the deck squats and rope climbs; it lets me physically shift into feeling and responding and going by instinct, not forcing and stressing or getting in my head about it — something I know an audience can detect. I see it as the key to going all in. Maybe you saw the tour where I exited the stage after "Live Like You Were Dying" by sliding on my knees, *Risky Business*-style, under the stage's massive video screen? In a moment like that, I'm so fully invested in what I'm doing, physically, mentally, and emotionally, there's no hesitation. My mind and my body are working together, translating sparks of inspiration into action, and I'm going for it — no hesitation.

I don't know what your experience is, but it sure makes it a good time for me.

My visualization ritual has trained me to pay attention to what's happening in my body at a keener level than I otherwise would, and to become more efficient with my energy and effort. It's helped me take ownership of my life by showing me how much control I hold over feeling how I want to feel, and creating the results I want to create. Bringing what I imagined in advance into reality helps me understand the extraordinary power of the mind, and how much better everything in life goes when you consciously choose to put your attention on your mental and physical states and notice every detail, not get lost in distraction and irrelevant thoughts. It's also taught me the difference between being halfway invested in something and giving it your all.

How does this apply to a fitness practice? Simple. Harness your mind's full potential to direct your attention onto what you're doing in the moment, and it will directly translate into physical effort, helping you work harder and better and perform beyond what you ever thought was possible. The way to do this is to become fully engaged in whatever kind of movement you're doing. I call this "dropping into deep focus" and it's the third

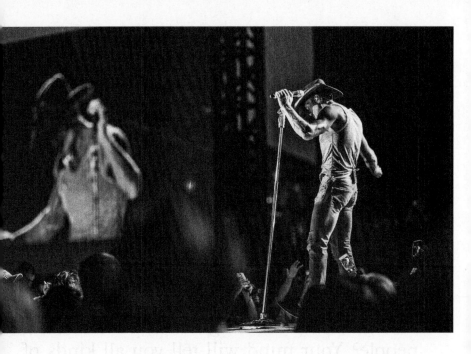

D in the mental tool kit — the apex of the pyramid that you can start to play with after you've connected to drive and discipline. Once you've got the habit for exercising going, and discipline in place, you'll free up some of the energy for going deeper, and starting to — note I say *starting to!* — master your practice. It's a lifelong effort to be able to stay in that apex of deep focus without wandering off mentally, and some days you won't be anywhere near it, but even the first steps toward it make a difference. As you get better at staying *in* what you're doing, this mental engagement helps you take your physical performance and your results to the next level.

You Must Be Present to Win

Have you ever gone for a run where you started out a little halfhearted, kept toggling between a jog and a walk every few minutes, then forgot to do the push-ups or crunches you'd promised yourself you'd do at the end? Or focused a little too much on the TV screen attached to the elliptical machine until your legs slowed down and you stopped breaking a sweat? Or gone to a class you'd signed up for only partly enthused, got your gear on as slow as molasses, then spent half the time shooting the shit with other people? Your mind will tell you all kinds of things. *I'm a little low energy today, I should take it easy.* Or, *I should talk to that person for a minute, I don't want to be rude.*

But if you're honest with yourself, what's really happening is that you're tap-dancing on the surface of your workout. You're dodging full commitment and only giving 50 percent of yourself, max, to the task at hand — and that might be a generous estimate. Sure, you get the workout done and strike it off your to-do list, but did you really get what you came for? There's no way around it. Working out is a kind of a *you get out what you put in* equation. Put 50 percent of yourself into it, you get 50 percent or less of the benefits.

We've all done it — I'm no stranger to this weakness. Sometimes my mind is deeply *in* the workout, and other times it's just shuffling around the edges. But I've earned a few nuggets of wisdom from attending my own school of hard knocks, and chief among them is that there's a night-and-day difference between when I'm mentally locked in and giving my all to my fitness regime and when I get complacent or distracted during my workouts. If I go through the motions on autopilot, or if my mind is simply elsewhere, focused not on the physical activity at hand but on the day's to-do list or something I'm stressed out about, the workout doesn't have the same effect. I don't feel as strong, integrated, or fluid because when I fail to connect the mental and physical in the moment and dig deep, I don't engage my whole body and stop working to the edge of my capacity, which means although I'm maintaining myself, I start to *lose* my edge. Movements that normally feel doable get harder, and it takes more effort to get momentum. If I phone it in for too many weeks in a row, I can even become a liability to myself, recruiting power from weak spots not strong ones or missing the physical cues that could be telling me I'm risking strain or injury. Maybe more important, my mental state after the workout isn't as sharp. There's a carryover effect from being distracted in the workout — it leads to being distracted everywhere else. I'm more anxious and susceptible to getting stressed. Getting sloppy in my fitness practices makes me start getting sloppy in life.

Luckily there's a flip side to this. When my head is fully engaged in what I'm doing and I'm truly focused, the positive results proliferate. Any motion you do can be done with full engagement or partial: Take a Bear Crawl, which is an animal-flow exercise of moving across the floor semi-inverted on hands and feet to build strength, mobility, and control. If you do it with full attention and engagement from head to toe, you'll be developing coordination, hip flexibility, and shoulder strength, and toning up your midback while releasing the tension and compression that builds up in your spine from sitting on your butt too long. With that deeper focus, you improve your skills at crawling and get better at speeding across the floor. You also get a fantastic, massage-style release. Do it lackluster, however, and your Bear Crawl becomes a mild cardio exercise that gets you from A to B, and that's it.

When we developed our TRUMAV gym we actually built a part of the programming around honing mental focus; the TRU-POWER workouts, which require passing a preliminary fitness test to join, are intense group workouts that make you work harder than you think you can, for longer. The logic behind this leap? We want to challenge you to overcome mental blocks. You are stronger than you think you are. That's a powerful lesson for life. Pushing yourself with any kind of challenge expands your physical limits and deepens your mental reserves.

When I fully engage my mind as I engage in intense physical activity — kind of like a skier dropping into a big line on a wild, untracked mountain, with no looking back and no questions — I feel the effects long after the workout is over. I feel more connected to myself, like I cleared out some of the static and noise inside or cleaned the windows to let more light in. As I move through the day, I'm more aware of my feelings or frustrations as they happen, better able to stay calm and neutral in the face of problems, and less triggered or reactive as a result. Bruce Lee said, "Concentration is the root of all the higher abilities in man." Tweak that quote to include *woman* as well as *man,* and I wholeheartedly agree. And we all know how Bruce honed his concentration. It wasn't by playing online Scrabble.

It's taken me a while to get to this point, but I've come to see being present to the whole experience of working out as a missing link to overall health and well-being. It's a training ground, a daily practice that teaches you to shift from being pushed and pulled by everything going on "out there" to what's really going on "in here." It helps you unplug from the whirlwind around you, with its flying debris of information and drama, and get plugged in to how you're feeling and functioning from the inside out. The reality's starting to land about the dire consequences of being surrounded by never-ending stimulation and the temptation to check our phones scores of times per day: we're getting more anxious without knowing why, becoming reactive and quick to take offense. We're falling into depression and losing sleep, not to mention losing connection with each other, and finding it hard to feel fulfillment from slower-paced things, or follow complex, nuanced ideas. It might sound too good to be true, but by directing your attention inward in a workout and anchoring it in for twenty minutes or thirty or more, refusing to let it wander off when it inevitably tries to do, you stake a stand: You start to take your mind back.

It's not like you'll be able to do this perfectly each time, but even chipping away at the goal and trying, then trying again, to focus your attention on the physical moment, makes a noticeable difference. You start a practice of becoming more present and then to how you're feeling and thinking about your body. You become more present to yourself. Over time this practice helps you become more present to those you care about, and eventually helps you radiate more *presence* — a state of calm, confident, inner strength — that just feels good to be around and makes other people want to engage with you, too. If you've ever managed to meditate successfully — a future goal of mine — you might already know this feeling. In a weird way, moving fast and with effort can offer some of the same benefits as sitting still and "not efforting," as the master meditators teach. Both have the potential to help you step out of the high-speed lane everyone's driving in today — too fast, too stressed, and overly consumed with just "getting there" — and into a different state entirely, where you take in more of your surroundings, get more out of the journey, and give a hell of a lot more attention and compassion to your fellow travelers on the road.

I Go Where I Look

So, if all these goods are up for grabs, why does it sometimes feel so hard to fully focus on a workout or even a simple walk and quiet the nagging chatter in our minds?

It partly comes down to the fact that the brain wants to conserve energy. It's not a big fan of exertion or pushing out of comfort mode and into a higher-octane state. *Why do that?* it says. *You're just wasting precious energy!* So it'll make anything *but* the physical challenge at hand seem super compelling, even addicting. *Look left — the TV's reporting breaking news! Look right — that person is way fitter than you! Look down — I bet work has e-mailed you and they need an answer now!* There's nothing that will tempt you to change the channel on what you're doing — or hit pause entirely — like asking your body to perform harder than normal.

Which makes working out today extra tricky. It's a circus out there! Gyms buzz with music and screens. The device you use to play music or stream an audio workout will also let the outside world into your precious exercise time one ping at a time if you're not on top of it. There's always something else to read or watch to stay smarter and more informed — so why not do double duty and catch up on media while you climb that elliptical mountain? And the excuses go on for multitasking through exercise, just like we multitask through life. But you have to be careful. Are you actually adding something of value or are you grooving in a pattern that when things get hard or uncomfortable, you can check out to someplace or something else?

One of my favorite sayings is "I go where I look." If you look down and get caught in distraction or comparison or endless bad news, that's where you go — down and stuck. If you check your phone between sets or take sly selfies at the weight rack, it doesn't just disrupt your personal effort, it sabotages any chance of achieving a sense of flow, it disconnects you from your body, and if you're exercising in a gym, it also drags down everyone else in the room. It's like throwing a rock into a window — it fractures the collective commitment. And it's a mirror of something bigger. If you're not comfortable being alone with yourself, just moving, breathing, and sweating, you're probably not comfortable being alone with yourself at all.

But maybe there's another reason you resist digging deep and giving your all. Maybe locking in fully to your body brings things *too* into focus, like how far away you currently feel from where you want to be or how dissatisfied you are with the shape you're in today. Ever heard the Keith Whitley song "I Never Go Around Mirrors"? It can be like that — you don't want to see your own reflection too clearly, so only having half your attention on the task seems like it'll make the whole task easier.

It won't. My fitness practice and my music career have served me that lesson in spades: There's no way to perform at your full potential if you're only partly there. Whether you're gripped by FOMO or wrapped in a funk of self-loathing — which we all have at times — you have to grab back control and outwit the part of yourself that says it doesn't want to be doing all this effort-and-sweat stuff. In my experience, the way through the awkward parts when you're not liking what you're seeing in the studio mirror or when you keep wanting to change the channel away from what you're seeing starts by doing the opposite of checking out: Get into your body by doing some of the tension-releasing techniques outlined in chapter 3. Start with a few minutes of active breathing — it'll melt some of the steely resistance you're feeling. Then if you're still at odds with yourself, take a few minutes to foam roll or release tension physically so you start feeling more comfortable to be in your body. Then practice acceptance: Look yourself in the eye, accept where you are starting from today, and give those thoughts of how you used to be or what else you could be doing right now over to some imaginary keeper for a while. Tell yourself you'll come back to them later. Now you're ready to *go where you look* in a bold and positive way: Look up at the horizon. See an imaginary finish line farther out than you ordinarily might. Remember your reason and passions that you hopefully wrote down if you were doing your homework! Now relax and have some faith in your body; the effort that will get you stronger and fitter than you are currently is well within reach.

Being fully engaged and present during your workout doesn't mean you have to be a master of mindfulness in everything you do. It just means that you focus as much of your attention and energy as possible on the physical task at hand. It also means keeping your attention on the physical experience even when it gets uncomfortable or hard. To do that, it helps to know your own tendencies: Why, where, and how do I check out instead of paying attention to what's going on inside?

Paying attention in this way has taught me a lot about myself, and one of my greatest lessons has been to temper my instinct to "go big." Because that's always been my default setting: Getting fast, agile, and strong has been my way of exorcising whatever stress I held through sheer manic effort. I'm one of the weird folks who don't have an issue seeing a hard workout through — I'll stick it out even if it almost floors me. The problem with this approach is that while the head rush drowns out any self-defeating inner voices, it can also drown out important messages from my body. The stress fractures in my foot that I got more than once and the dehydration that came from mixing long-haul plane travel with extra-tough workouts? Those were my teachers showing me I hadn't yet learned to listen. What can I say? Sometimes when you're a hammer all you see is nails — you hit hard and hit harder until someone takes the hammer out of your hand.

Hurtling through things is my Kryptonite — which Roger quickly saw when we met. I couldn't hold a yoga pose for more than two beats without getting antsy. And learning to do a martial-arts kick the way he likes to teach it — which is to break it down to the smallest detail, step by step — made me crazy at first. But I'm finally learning that Go Big has a brother called Go Deep, and if I slow my roll and bring my full attention to the exercise at hand — whether it's a walk, a dive, a strength-building circuit or a mix of yoga and mobility — I become a better athlete by feeling every movement from the inside out. It's not so much mind over matter as it is mind *into* matter. I also get a lot more out of less, like with those eight really good reps that use every muscle fiber deliberately instead of the twenty-two my ego wants to do, pushing to hit a high number for the sake of it but with sloppy form.

I'm also enabling myself to do this for longer, because a mentally engaged athlete is a safe athlete, one who notices when he or she is about to pull a hamstring by doing one set of deadlifts too many or is verging on tweaking a back muscle because their core isn't tight. Or who actually stops for a second and realizes, *Something's off. If I push myself today, this tickle in my throat might turn into a real cold* — and then changes the plan to something less intense. One of my great lessons has been that intensity comes in many different forms. Pushing yourself so hard that your T-shirt looks like you just wore it in the shower is one version, while

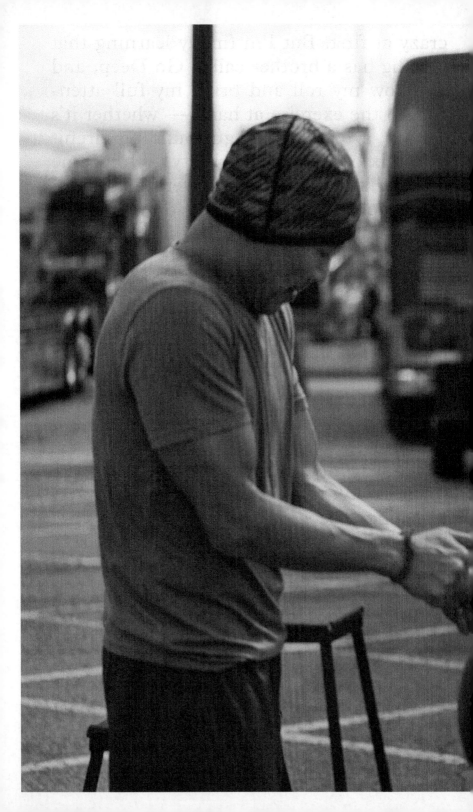

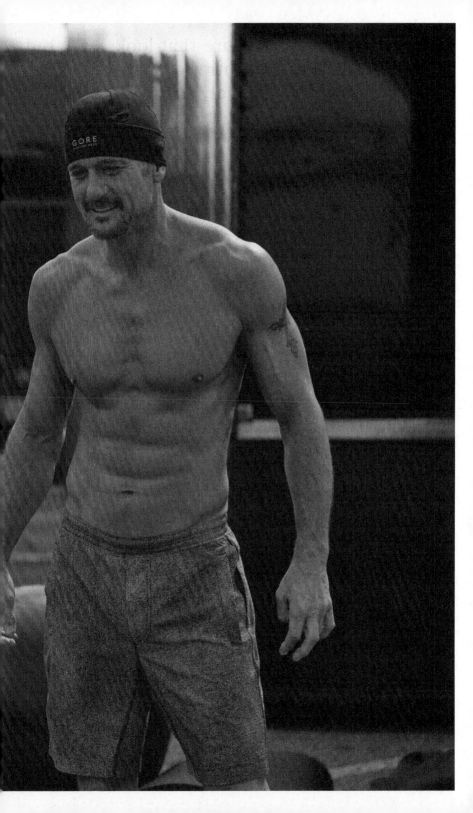

holding a static posture that looks easy but requires deep concentration and coordination is another. In fact, such poses help to rewire your brain and create body awareness — the ability to tune in very specifically to where your body is in space and appreciate how minute adjustments improve your form — as well as develop "muscle memory," in which your muscles become familiar with movement. When you hone these abilities — something that can only happen when you integrate deep focus into your workouts — you'll be able to learn new forms of fitness faster. That's because you're not only *feeling* more familiar with them, you're also literally building them into being by strengthening the pathways of signaling in the brain and nervous system that help you engrain them.

I won't lie: Growing deeper focus has taken a hell of a resolve because I'm undoing years of thinking that harder and faster always equals better. It might not be the same for you. Perhaps your big lesson is that your body actually has what it takes to deliver more strength, speed, or stamina — if you can just guide your mind to drop the resistance and stop thinking that it can't. Either way, consider that there may be another angle to view fitness from: It's not always the difficulty of the workout you do, or how polished it looks in the mirror, or how advanced you are compared to others; it's the way you engage in your workout and the attitude you bring to it that matters, and maybe matters more than anything else.

I can lose my A-game attitude in a heartbeat, just like you can. I get off rhythm when I'm on the road for a while then off it all of a sudden, or when things at home need tending to, like someone I love being sick or one of my girls stepping into a new phase of life and needing extra dad-help. So I've developed a bag of tricks to dip into at the first sign of flagging. Sometimes I'll use them to just make it through the first twelve minutes of a workout so I can build all-important momentum. Other times they're what I use to make it through the third round of a circuit, when everything seems much harder than in the first two rounds, or to maintain my starting pace in the last five laps of a fifty-lap swim. Whatever the task at hand, dropping into deep focus is a practice of *making it count.* If something's worth doing and spending your precious time on, you might as well get the most out of it. It'll give a turbocharge to whatever you do — from the simplest exercise to the most complex.

1 ADJUST YOUR ATTITUDE. If I'm ever getting slack, I repeat the credo *It's easier to keep fit than get fit.* And that's not just a catchphrase. Anytime I've gotten injured or taken too much time off, it's a lot more work to get back on the wagon than it would have been to just stay on it. I've learned to embrace the spike of fear I feel around stopping for too long; it kicks in when I'm getting complacent to remind me I've put so much work into getting where I am that losing it will be like going back to the beginning. It does the job of steering me straight. That said, once I start exercising, all negative self-talk is banned; that's shown to impede performance. Telling yourself you suck at what you're doing is like spraying an extinguisher on your drive. It kills the passion to try harder.

2 DO A RUN-THROUGH. I seal in my workout plan with a short visualization before sleeping. The whole nine yards, from picturing myself getting out of bed and suited up, to cooling down and grabbing water at the end and how my body will feel after I successfully finish. This whole process can be done quickly and at high speed, touching on the key points only. But it's effective: It makes it all a lot closer and more real, like I've done the sketch for the artwork I want to create.

3 SET UP SOME WALLS. One of the reasons working out with a community is so powerful is that the group focus is like a bubble that that keeps all distractions out. If you don't have that yet, go somewhere where people are focused on working out — even a running track at the local high school will do. Joining a culture of fitness automatically sets you up for greater success. Wherever you exercise, be sure to lay down some boundaries to keep intrusion out. I'll confess to watching the news during my early morning treadmill walks. Staying informed is important to me, and that's my time to catch up with world affairs. But once the workout starts, it's good-bye to all that. No phones, no e-mail, no checking anything but my own physical technique and form — and we shoot the shit only in the rest periods between rounds. The world will conspire to find you, so it's about being super deliberate with your choices. If the deal for stepping away from your desk or your caregiving role is that you remain on call to others, set a timer to a reasonable increment of time, at least fifteen minutes away, and pledge to be N/A 'til it goes off. And if there's no way to get an hour uninterrupted, make your workout a focused twenty minutes.

On that note, if you're using an app of some kind to guide or track your workout — both of which can be a terrific way to get focused — close all other apps so that nothing comes in to break your concentration. I wager it's worth setting up an old-school stereo if using your phone for music proves too distracting. But what about making sure that some of your workouts are 100 percent tech- and noise-free? It might feel odd at first to exercise without music, but you'll soon be surprised how much your senses come alive, taking in the world around you or noticing more about how your body's functioning. Silence is the starting point for finding more depth.

4 SCAN YOURSELF BEFORE YOU START. My fitness sensei Roger

teaches that checking in with how you feel on *every level* before working out helps you train intelligently. He likes to say, "Always balance your intensity with physical, mental, and emotional stability. If you're feeling solid physically but you're angry and upset, it can lead to wanting to escape and overdoing it; if you're mentally exhausted and push yourself too hard, your coordination and perception of space can be off. That's when injuries occur." I've tried to use a workout as a venting mechanism for a pissed-off mood many a time. It works occasionally, but often I come out feeling worse. I figure that's because I haven't actually reckoned with what's going on inside — I've just tried to steamroll over it with tire flips and medicine ball slams. I'm learning to take a moment of reckoning before I start and acknowledge my demons, then tell them I'll attend to them later, after I've purged the stress and tension they're creating. This sets me up to look the deeper issues square in the eye with a clear head. It may not make my workout a seated mindfulness practice, but it gets me a little closer to knowing myself, and making a better choice about what to do next.

And no matter what mood I'm in, I always look at my mantras on my gym wall and lock into a phrase that captures the mood and results I want. *Be relentless!* on one day; *killer workout: killer show* on another. That single word or phrase can even be repeated at a rhythm to crowd other thoughts — such as *I don't want to do this!* or *That's enough, let's call it* — out of your mind. If mantras work to take meditators deeper into their experience on the cushion, they can also work in the gym to override the monkey-mind chatter. Try it.

5 **INHALE. EXHALE.** Faith has been saying it for years: *Breathe.* She's way smarter than I am. I had to train myself to do it as I upped my regimen because holding or restricting my breath was a pattern that was hard to break. Good breathing patterns are a must in order to brace your midsection and protect all the muscles there when you lift weights. Breath is also the quickest pathway inward for reining in your roving attention — it guides your mind into your body. Sound too simple? Give it a whirl. As you warm up, notice the sensation of air moving into your nose, down

your windpipe, and into your lungs; feel your ribs expanding open and stretching your back wider. Really feel how it feels, without rushing past it. Then keep returning to the breath throughout your workout. This one trick can redirect your attention from outward to inward in a nanosecond. And it helps you discover something so easily overlooked but so important to overall health and happiness: the realization that *Wow, my body feels really good right now.*

6 TIME IT. If you're having trouble digging deep, try putting a timer into the mix. Exerting yourself in intervals, like forty-five seconds on/ fifteen off, will stop you waffling like nobody's business. Forty-five seconds feel a lot longer than you think they will and fifteen seconds a lot shorter. Stepping up to that intensity demands mental focus. Try making your grocery list when the clock's ticking on your burpees: You can't. Similarly, AMRAP (As Many Rounds As Possible) workouts challenge you to do as many reps of certain exercises as you can in a set period of minutes. If you have even the smallest competitive bone in your body, you'll want to hit a high number, and that number gives you a focal point. Beating your previous times split on the rower or a mile on the treadmill can have similar effect. Group workouts (in person and now even online) that use a heart rate monitor and show who's working hardest can also laser focus you on the task at hand. Research shows that higher intensity exercise may burn fat successfully partly *because* of the focus required: To get through it, you end up using more effort and recruiting more muscles. If you're working out with others, there's the obvious: Competing against each other for fastest times will harness your mind and set it to win. In our tour workouts, we pair up to compete for time on weighted-sled relays, giving it our all to push the sled X yards faster than the next guys. You'll see examples of simple timed workouts in chapter 6.

7 **HIT REFRESH.** Autopilot exercising means it's time to add variety and get a new part of my mind engaged in learning. The best way to do this is adding the challenge of mastering something new. I'm grateful for being in the position where I can purchase new toys to test me and my workout crew. Our

most recent addition to the TRUMAV traveling trailer are mace clubs — heavy, ancient-warrior-looking implements for advanced training that you swing (carefully) around your body to build core power and rotational strength. Learning to do this with really good movement patterns takes concentration; you don't want to just start throwing a mace club wildly. Even without gear, adding challenge could be as simple as turning everyday pull-ups into harder-for-you chin-ups. Or maybe it's trying a new sport or fitness practice entirely for a few weeks — adopting what the Zen masters call "beginner's mind" and showing up with absolutely no experience to move in a completely different way than you ever have before. Find something that piques your curiosity and tests your ability, and getting mentally reengaged will come easier than plugging away at your old standard routine, stuck in a rut.

8 USE THE NO-QUIT TRICK. The moment I sense I want to bail on a session, I tell myself, *If I do a little bit more now, tomorrow will be easier.* Haven't made it to twelve-minute mark? *Do a little more now.* Flagging at the nineteen-minute mark? *Do a little more now.* It's about breaking the macro goal of being healthy and strong for life into its smallest and most immediate increment: Just commit to right now. Does this actually make tomorrow's workout easier? I think it does because there's no momentum lost and the habit stays nicely sealed in. Plus, if I can even do one more good rep today than yesterday, it's like throwing myself a bone. It ups my drive to continue.

A similar trick applies if I wake up totally uninspired. I tell myself, *If I work out today, I can take tomorrow off.* Setting up the possibility is a kind of soothing balm for my mind, it takes the edge off the quitting notion. Once I've gotten warm and moving, my body remembers why this is a habit and taking tomorrow off doesn't usually feel as appealing. That said, if I do wake up the next morning and want the day off, I honor my pledge. I feel fine about skipping, knowing that the next day, it's back on, same time, same place. And there's no beating myself up about it. I did what I said I would.

Getting older and hopefully wiser shifts your priorities around. You go from wanting to achieve some kind of perfect status to appreciating the process of moving toward your goals. More than a few philosophical writings teach that it's not reaching the destination that brings joy and satisfaction; it's working toward it and engaging in the process of learning the lessons to get there, of growing and evolving and building self-esteem. This is what helps you become a master of your body, someone who starts to know intuitively what you need today, when you need to step up, when you need to dial down, and how to get to each place. When you train your mind to go deep, you'll notice more of what you're doing as you're doing it. Get into the process and be awake to how everything feels from the inside out. That's how even the most stripped-down exercise session — a walk in the fall forest, a cold swim in the summer lake — becomes something to remember, a piece of the story of how you lived. And then moving your body becomes something else entirely; not just a healthy habit, but a way of being that makes life feel deeper and more richly lived.

Part III
Train the Body

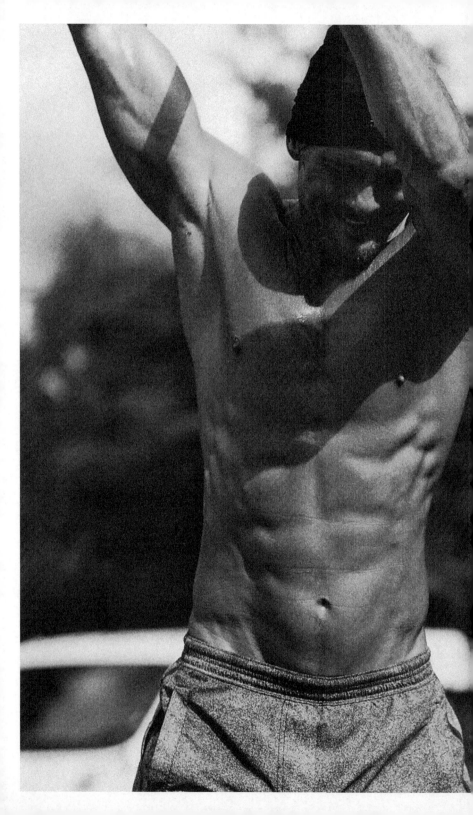

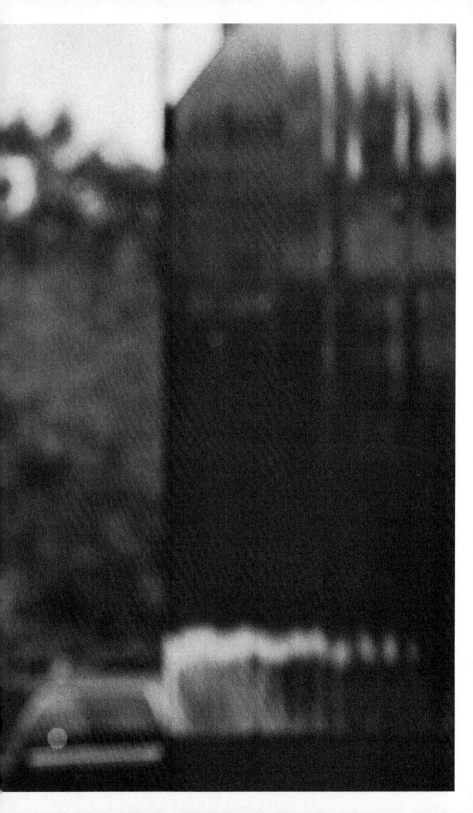

So we've got the basic concepts laid out and the case is made. Working out is about more than honing a hard body; it's about building resilience and releasing stress, growing grit, and touching grace. Now comes the hard part — actually getting it done. And I want to be honest: Getting it done doesn't come easy. It requires giving it everything you've got.

That doesn't mean that this journey is for black diamond experts only. Making the choice to get healthier, fitter, and stronger starts with a commitment to going all in, and that's within everyone's reach. If you have the guts for it, that is.

Truth be told, there are myriad routes to the destination of health and vitality, and almost any of them will generate some physical benefit. But what all of them have in common is that they can only deliver the benefits if you start doing them, and then keep doing them, not just for a week, a month, or a season, but through all the seasons of your life. Consistency is key.

Having access to gyms, trainers, or fancy technology may be part of your journey, and it may not. There is no one "right" way to do this, and getting fit doesn't have to cost a lot of money. In fact, one study of people who'd kept significant weight off for over two years highlighted something interesting: Those who are most successful at sustaining healthy lifestyles for the long term aren't necessarily the ones with the most resources. They're the ones who have developed a sense of ownership by landing on a way of healthy living that works uniquely well for them; over time, they have honed their best way of eating and exercising that suits their bodies, lifestyles, and interests. They've found what fits.

To that end, my goal is to inspire and guide you with what I've discovered works well. I want to help you get to where the "right" choice and the "fun" choice merge and it starts to feel better to do the hard thing than not to do it. This is a powerful junction; it's where you gain momentum and the effort becomes a little easier. You find your groove, and making healthy choices starts to become automatic. When you're in this groove, you can spend less energy on the motivation to get going and grind through the work and spend more of it on getting creative, having fun with physical activity, exploring your full potential, and really doing *you*.

The best way to get this groundwork down? Follow a well-tested course, mapped out by a guide who's been up and down the mountain a few times, even if not always completely smooth. I don't have a perfect formula for making it easy 24/7. My own route involved a few mishaps. But with trial and error I've forged a trusty set of tools that I rely on day in and day out. And I'm excited to share them here with you.

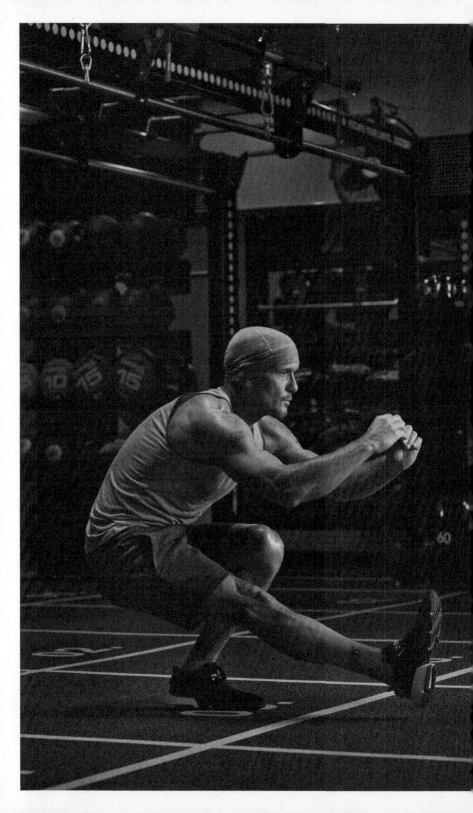

CHAPTER 6
GET MOVING

What you'll find in this chapter is a simplified approach to fitness inspired by my own journey. It's a program that anyone can benefit from and everyone can follow no matter their starting point. And you're going to go at your own pace — it wouldn't be smart to throw you into uphill sprints with a wrestling bag or unsupervised heavy kettlebell swings on Day 1; that's just a quick way to injure yourself if you're not ready for those kinds of drills (though if you are ready, I'm happy to show you how I do these exercises!).

Rest assured, there is still plenty of work to do before any of that occurs (and that's with a caveat — it might never occur, because as awesome as I personally find uphill wrestling-bag runs, they're not for everyone and not a prerequisite for health). On page 342, you'll find workouts that are similar to the ones my bandmates and I do on tour, but I encourage you to take your time to get there. Read through what comes first, because believe it or not there's a method to this madness.

My route to get there has been my own spin on functional fitness. *Functional fitness* is a phrase that's been widely used over the last ten or so years. I see it as a style of training that works the whole body to perform optimally by strengthening its capacity to do the motions you need in everyday life: squatting down and lifting up boxes; carrying heavy bags; pushing around furniture; bursting into a quick sprint to catch a bus or train. All stuff that, if you don't train for it, can give you a swift message that you're not in shape. (Have you ever lifted something from the floor at an odd angle and felt a searing twinge in your body? That's the kind of message I mean.) Functional fitness as I see it also aims to *keep you functional* for as long as possible. It might seem banal to talk about training to lift things off the floor of your home or pull something off the top shelf in the garage, but believe me, you don't know what you have until it's gone. It pays off a hundredfold tomorrow to put effort into maintaining and developing your capacity for movement today.

And then there's the obvious: Functional fitness is FUN. It takes training out of the

266

realm of clanking machines into a free-form space (like our Gorilla Yard) full of different objects to play with, pushes you to move fast and keep going harder, and allows you to throw things around and occasionally howl it out like a wild animal. And hopefully, like anything else that tests you but you know is momentary, it gives you a laugh or two on the way.

Here's a twist you may not expect: In my way of seeing it, a daily physical training practice *may* be a source of meaning and joy to you, something that becomes core to who you are and what makes you tick. But I think it's important to say right now, equally, it may not — and that's okay, too. What I want you to see is that regular training *sets you up for a more supported experience in your whole life — whatever that involves and whatever has the most meaning to you.* It could mean hoisting grandkids onto your back or leap-frogging alongside them, today or in the future. It could mean entering a muddy Spartan race where you climb obstacles and run triumphantly through mud, or learning a new sport or activity you've always wanted to try. It could mean leaping off a stage in a moment of insanity and flying over outstretched hands. It's about being ready for anything.

I want any and all of that to be possible for you, because whatever you end up doing with your well-prepared body, it all comes down to the same principle: You train so that your body can handle the demands you place on it without a negative cost. How "demanding" you choose to go is up to you, your personality, your interests — or as I've experienced, your career choice. That will vary widely. But what doesn't vary is that none of us can afford to overlook maintaining the natural-born capacity for movement that we came in with, and once you get the taste for it, you just may want to go beyond maintaining it, and really getting in there to grow it, hone it, and discover how much more capacity is currently untapped. We all get older, we all face similar stressors and pressures just by virtue of living a twenty-first-century lifestyle. It's up to us to protect what we have!

To pull that off, it's better not to chase "fast-food fitness" — jumping straight into the hardest, most intense or complex new thing that promises an instant fix or overnight transformation. Just like fast food comes with a price, so does that approach. There's a secret that's not talked about enough when it comes to training — the amount of strains and injuries that come as a result of going too big too soon. What I want to help you do is avoid that by building the foundation from the bottom up.

Our bodies are the instruments we were given at birth and, boy, are they incredible. They have so much potential that we barely even explore. And when we don't use them enough, they fall out of tune and all sorts of discomforts start to build up. You might know some of them: an achy, tight back, or soreness and stiffness in the shoulders and hips; body fat accumulating in the midsection. Even things like skin problems, poor digestion, anxiety and depression, food cravings, and low sex drive can be related to the imbalances that arise when you get sedentary and stuck. When these things start to happen, it can screw with your head. You can start to think your instrument is flawed. I want to show you that so many of those symptoms result from a lack of playing your instrument. You skipped practice a few too many days, months, or years, is all. And it's well within reach to get back in the swing of things and find your own song again!

Equally, I want to help you see how important it is to respect your instrument and treat it carefully. It can play extraordinary music — it can even get you to the fitness equivalent of a rock star solo that has a stadium on its feet — but not if you trash it in the first few months of playing it.

Of course, not everyone wants to take playing music to the same level, and not everyone wants to train the same way. Getting to the place where you stop traffic with your torso probably isn't a bucket list wish unless you *really* love working out and will religiously choose the lettuce wrap. In fact, while changing or refining your physique is a great motivation — it might be one of the first "whys" on your list of reasons and is a fun, inspiring goal for some people — it's also powerful to flip this perspective around and consider physical transformation from a different approach. Why not start your fitness journey by asking, *How can I best serve my body so I experience ease of movement and little discomfort, can physically accomplish all the things I want to do, am consistently releasing stress, am continuously growing and discovering what I can do, even as I get older and as I experience all the stages of my life?* Then trust that as a result of this process of discovery, if you commit and stay on track, and don't get in a rut or cheat yourself of putting in the effort, your body composition will change. The change in your physique becomes the gift you receive from staying in the process rather than the goal you're chasing.

Similarly, here's another mind hack to help give you perspective: *You only need to be slightly stronger and more mobile than the activities you have to do or want to do.* What that means is that not everyone has to train like an MMA fighter preparing for the championship bout. Nevertheless, don't dismiss the level of capability you need simply for daily living. If you're a parent, can you carry your melting-down child, his backpack, and your groceries, and get out of a deluge or even a dangerous situation quickly? If your job requires lifting boxes or stocking shelves, can you lift and swivel safely under load? If you're a gardener, can you cart bags of potting soil and push wheelbarrows full of gravel across your yard, then dig ditches without strain? These are no small feats, and they are worthy of preparation.

Roger and I talk about this stuff when he's not torturing me with Chair Pose. He's arrived at this philosophy after years of competitive martial-arts fighting and helping on-screen performers quickly learn to inhabit their bodies in a whole new way for action roles. And, now in his fifties, he looks at fitness very differently than he did in his twenties. I confess I'm not yet fully there myself, but I love this way of looking at changing your body because it tempers the temptation to get rigid or obsessive; it's not focused 100 percent on the external. It's recognizing that the body is something to be not mastered or perfected, but rather befriended and supported and encouraged to evolve so it never gets stagnant or stuck. Especially, as Roger likes to say, "If you're an old dog, it's important to be able to teach your body new tricks!"

True fitness is also acknowledging that part of being human is moving through all kinds of life phases. There will be times when you're looking like a badass — when you welcome a camera pointed at your beach body because you damn well want this saved for posterity — and other times when it all gets a little less so. Maybe you're studying for exams, or just became a parent, or started a business, or must look after an aging family member, or are working through a health challenge. Yet even when those phases occur, if you're doing something for your body daily, no matter how small, and doing your best to tend to its needs when you feel areas of concern, it's okay. The journey involves curves in the road and there will be times when you can just do the basics and times when you can dial it up all the way. The cumulative effect will be that you do a great job maintaining your vehicle over time just as the manufacturer intended, and you get a great drive out of it, putting a lot of miles on the odometer.

When I get in tour shape, it's about dialing it up. Way up! I hear it all the time: *What you do is so hard core, Tim!* And my answer is that yes, sometimes it is, because one of my personal goals is pretty specific. I set myself at the task of operating as a high-level performer in a fairly high-stakes game. There's a lot riding on me as an artist and I want to meet that pressure by showing up at my peak of health and fitness. So my version of the best shape of my life is relative to the everyday demands I face. My "personal best" benchmarks are set high because I'm essentially training for a championship game — on show in a big way with a lot of people on my team and my business depending on my performance.

Your version of the best shape of your life will be unique to you and the demands of your life. You don't have to hold yourself to the standard of an elite performer or athlete. Instead, keep connecting to what your life requires of you right now. Your personal best is likely different from your neighbor's and is probably different from your personal best ten years ago — and I don't necessarily mean it's lower today, because very often as you get older, you get wiser and feel more dedicated to pursue a personal dream than you did before. Your personal best also might look different from day to day. Some days it might mean pushing hard, breathing hard, causing your muscles to tremble with exertion . . . other days it might be rolling out on a foam roller, releasing tension, and breathing deeply and slowly.

To me that's what fitness is — a well-rounded approach that's fed by a certain amount of body intelligence and backed by the skills that come from learning basic movements well. It's also about stoking the physical energy and the mental drive to take care of yourself from one day to the next. Getting in good shape doesn't have to be rocket science, and there is plenty of time to add complexity and nuance. What I hope to do is help you put a simple framework in place to start finding your way there yourself.

WELL-ROUNDED FITNESS

These days it's become confusing to tackle the subject of getting fit. There is So. Much. Information. And everyone seems to want to persuade you their way is best! While it can be inspiring, it can also be overwhelming. You might look at the endless options available to you and think, *Where do I even start?*

I'm a firm believer that all types of movement and exercise are worthy and that anything you enjoy doing or that adds to your life should be celebrated. When it comes to moving, nothing is wrong; and as a nation we need to do a lot more of it. Even so, if you are seeking to increase your health and longevity, reverse the degenerative effects of a sedentary lifestyle, develop a total body strength that helps you move well in everything you do, and hone your physique to have less fat and more muscle, then you're going to want to have a strategy.

Let me explain. Have you ever gotten into doing one kind of physical activity as your source of exercise, and then stuck with it, maybe for years? Perhaps you do that because it's become your default "thing you do," or you like the place or people you exercise with. Or perhaps you're not sure how to add other dimensions to that plan. Maybe it looks like going to the gym, doing some cardio on a machine, then a few sets of crunches and mat work. Or maybe it's running a set number of miles per day or week. Perhaps it's yoga class regularly or maybe it's frequent golf. You feel good after you do these things, probably — there's no doubt they benefit body and mind — and if you're doing them consistently, congratulations!

You're one of a fairly small percentage of people who do have a regular exercise practice. But I have another question: Has your body changed shape significantly in ways that make you happy, and have you gotten stronger and more capable of handling everyday demands, and are you able to leap into a new recreation on vacation easily with nary a tweak, twinge, or uncoordinated wobble?

I'd bet that for most people, one or more of the above questions might generate a "no." They're not getting the full benefits they could from a more well-rounded approach, and they're missing key pieces of the total fitness puzzle. Roger calls single-track practice a "Damocles Sword." When you develop one set of skills, whether it's at an extremely high level like he did as a competitive fighter or even just at a recreational level, over time the same skills that make you good at something also take a toll because too much pressure is continuously exerted on specific parts of the body without restorative, counterbalancing practices from other types of movement. In addition, that approach often lacks the fundamental and very protective element of solid core strength achieved from training the whole body in an integrated way. Done the same way, year after year, a single-track practice tends to lead to wear and tear.

The alternative? A sustainable athleticism that lets you perform for the long term with more resiliency against stress and strain. I'm certainly not saying you shouldn't do the activities you love or that you shouldn't have goals of mastering certain sports or types of exercise, but just consider that it may not be a complete system on its own. My suggestion is to pull back the lens and look from a wider viewpoint. If you develop a baseline of well-rounded, total-body strength and fitness as your foundation and learn how to move from a strong core, you make your body your reliable rock. A strong core doesn't just mean having sexy abs; it is the central pillar that you build when you strengthen your whole midsection from diaphragm down to pelvis, in front and in back. It protects your spine, major joints, and even your brain. Then, you can bring that stable and powerful rock to the sport or activity that brings you joy. In other words, spend some time consistently developing well-rounded fitness, then let the sport or activity you love be *an expression of that fitness, not the way you get fit.* You'll not only bring a wholly upgraded version of yourself to that activity, you'll set yourself up to keep enjoying it well into your golden years.

This approach also applies if you haven't gotten in the groove with any particular physical activity yet, and even if doing regular physical activity at all feels like a stretch. Don't worry. The way we're going to get into this is as simple as it comes.

HOW A MAVERICK DOES IT

Until I landed on my current way of working out, I had more of what Roger affectionately called a good ol' boy workout style: a traditional gym workout using machines and benches to balance out the cardio stuff. It got me pretty fit and kept me fairly focused, though it got humdrum at times. When I started seeing this new type of exercise around called functional fitness, I had an "aha" moment. With its primal-style, full-body movements like lifting, hanging, and carrying, I loved that it looked a little lawless. It made sense to fuse cardio and strength training together in the same workout to get maximum bang for the buck, and I liked the "metabolic conditioning" drills that programmed short periods of effort followed by periods of rest to condition the energy systems of the body. Because a lot of the movements worked upper and lower body together and multiple joints at once, I could immediately see how hard the cardiovascular system would work and how the whole body had to function as one to maintain balance, coordination, and motor control. The exercises mimicked how humans actually *move* instead of isolating a body part at a machine, and it struck me how swinging a weighty sledgehammer overhead to hit a truck tire would not only develop a core of steel but also make a golf swing or tennis stroke unbeatable, as momentum drove up from the feet and through the whole body like lightning. Moving the body this way was retraining the neuromuscular system to wake up and work at a whole new level. Above all, it looked youthful, fluid, and animalistic to me — the three qualities I most wanted my body to have!

So I basically taught myself some of the moves I'd seen and started training this way. What I noticed pretty quickly was that all kinds of activities got better, from games of flag football with friends to moving onstage. Sprinting to score a touchdown felt turbocharged, and so did the endurance to make it through a whole show. The positive impact hit home in three small scenes that happened after starting this new routine.

In one, I'm working around my yard and go to yank a giant boulder off the ground without thinking. As I twist down to the left to hoist the weight of the rock at an off angle, slightly wobbly on one leg, I have a flash that this is the exact kind of maneuver that'll throw your back out. But, conditioned from the training sessions, my midsection braces as my glutes, hamstrings, and all the muscles of my trunk do the work and I'm stable as a tree as I hoist that thing from ground to truck bed. In another, I'm paddleboarding with my daughters and rocketing across the water with powerful, diagonal strokes that rotate my torso while my feet, ankles, knees, hips, and shoulders microadjust to every ripple and bounce. And in a third, I'm singing *"Real Good Man."* Charged on adrenaline, I drop into the one-legged pistol squat I've been practicing in workouts like a fiend, usually struggling to hold it but now nailing it and feeling I could hold it forever. My hours of conditioning and practice have seared the muscle memory into me and built the strength and flexibility required, and suddenly it feels easy. If you've ever worked on a pistol squat let me tell you — that's a triumph!

I've always followed the philosophy, *Be primed to get to your highest level at any moment.* This kind of training helped me get closer to that than I'd ever been before. It didn't hurt that my physique got leaner and more defined from boosting my metabolism and burning fat for longer while also building muscle through strength training.

When I met Roger, he evaluated the missing pieces in what I was doing, and helped me develop an approach that came closer to a complete system. Turned out, I was so excited about the speed and power aspects of my workouts that I hadn't put much attention on flexibility, pliability, or releasing the tightness that inevitably resulted from pushing hard. I was creating strong, dense muscles that were neither supple nor flexible, which was keeping me from that fluidity of movement I craved. And I wasn't taking time to consciously care for my joints and connective tissues through mobility exercises — connective tissues include the tendons that join muscles to bone, the ligaments that live inside joints and join bones together, and the fascia, the net of collagen fibers that surrounds all the muscles, bones, organs, nerves, and blood vessels, and keeps everything gliding when they touch rather than sticking with friction. That's what had me skewing toward the bulky "gym guy" look — where your tight body is impressive aesthetically but makes you walk like a robot. For someone who makes music to move to, robot-walk is a no-no.

I'm a hard nut to crack, but Roger put the pragmatic spin on things — since he's a few years older than I am, I can joke he's the wise elder. He says that workouts are constantly evolving and if you want to move well for longer, you want to make your workouts short, efficient, and not necessarily all-out each time. And you shouldn't seek to be the grittiest person in the room all the time, but one who balances grit with grace. Translation: Use your fitness practice to push your body to work hard (but not to exhaustion each time), and become a master of your movement by developing strength along with mobility, flexibility, and agility. Develop some body intelligence — connecting to your body and noticing what it's telling you — and the cumulative effect is that you begin to move fluidly and really enjoy being in your body. He made our workouts totally hybrid, with yoga moves and animal-flow moves mixed into the drills and showed us how slowing down a boxing punch to super-slow motion can teach you to make contact not from the hands, but all the way from the ground, transferring from foot to ankle to knee to hip to shoulders and out the arms. "In slow motion, a punch or kick should look like a dance," Roger says, with a nod to grace. "A good athlete knows how to move economically, efficiently, always in balance, and structurally always in alignment."

Together, we landed on a well-rounded approach that I call maverick functional fitness — a way of servicing the body daily that helps you perform better, look great, and have a lot of fun while doing it.

This style has been put to the test by the many people who've passed through our Team McGraw training camp with different levels of ability, interest, and desire for change. What most everyone has in common is a desire to burn fat and build lean muscle, improving body composition while taking care of our hearts and keeping our energy systems burning fuel nicely. We're also doing it to avoid wear and tear and feel younger for longer. But it's an inclusive approach that's not dogmatic. We say, *Take the parts of this that work for you.* Wendy, our backup singer, joins us for our mobility warm-up drills to open up her body, get everything loose and limber, and warm up her instrument before a show. She doesn't do the circuit workouts that follow, but she does some walking or brief cardio on a treadmill or elliptical instead.

Our drummer Shawn takes just one element of the approach. He likes to walk, and walk he does. A lot of it. If we're at an airport, Shawn finds a way to get miles of walking in during a layover. Strength training is not his thing, but he still makes it a priority to take care of his body and connect to himself each day, paying into his physical and mental health.

THE PYRAMID OF FITNESS

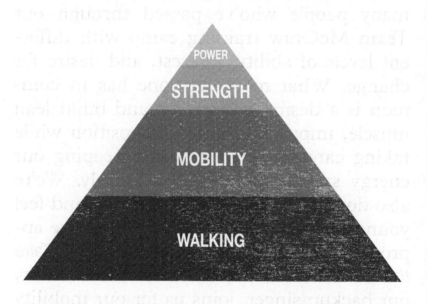

Just like we used a pyramid approach in our mental training, I think it's helpful to use a similar model when it comes to physical training — this time, with four layers that together help you build a super-solid state of health. The way I see it is that the first two layers help you get better "function" in your body — a terrific goal on its own. The second two layers step it up a notch in an effort to develop your actual "fitness." If your habits touch on all four levels, you develop a state of functional fitness where you get your best health and reap the highest physical and mental benefits. But what I really want to convey is that even the activity at the base of the pyramid has the potential to change your life. Don't look at this structure and think you have to do it all at once, right now. Start at the base level, get a habit down, let it help you love exercise, and if and when you're ready, look to the next level.

The first layer of the pyramid is *walking*. That's right, walking. The most natural of movements has so many benefits that doctors and researchers call it a panacea — a remedy for all difficulties. It is an exercise that humans evolved to do daily — scientists say that the act of walking helped to develop our advanced human brains — and conversely when we don't do it, we struggle and suffer. Purposeful walking, swinging arms in sync with your stride, gets your heart rate going moderately and helps restore natural breathing patterns. If done for at least thirty minutes a day, it can help to strengthen bones, lower blood pressure, reduce excess body fat, boost muscle power and endurance, and reduce the risk of heart disease, type 2 diabetes, osteoporosis, and some cancers while also reducing stress and anxiety and boosting outlook and mood. It helps keep the lymph system, part of the body's waste and toxin-removal system, working well. Walking demands you hike the hip up slightly in order to take each step; this small action is one of the first things you lose if you become sedentary, contributing to overall decline, so training it through daily walking is invaluable as you age.

Walking also improves posture, giving the spine and pelvis a chance to reset and letting all the postural muscles release compression and tension. It helps to *integrate the body* through the core, as opposite arms and legs work dynamically together in a similar way to our very first human movement, crawling. Every time you do this, you are literally reminding your nervous system how to function as a whole unit working together, which is vital not just for good health but also for safety, so you have greater coordination and more awareness of your body in space!

I get some of my clearest ideas when I'm walking — you know how babies take leaps in development when they learn to crawl? That phenomenon doesn't stop. Walking's "contralateral" pattern — left leg, right arm; right leg, left arm — helps the two hemispheres of the brain communicate and if done vigorously, helps the brain produce new cells in the area responsible for spatial awareness and memory. It literally grows your brain bigger and even better, and significantly helps stave off age-related mental decline and dementia: Two miles of walking per day has been shown to help lower the risk of these afflictions by up to 60 percent. (Other moderately aerobic exercises like swimming and biking have similar protective effect . . . and by the way, performing the same two miles briskly has been shown to improve sexual function in men.) Walking after you eat also helps your blood sugar stay better regulated (which might be why there's a longstanding tradition of taking an after-dinner stroll).

For all these reasons, walking is the gateway to longevity and a basic state of health. It's a low-impact activity that anyone can start and a great choice if you've been inactive or are overweight. Where running can put injury-causing load on deconditioned joints and tissues, and if done to excess can have a degenerative effect, walking tends to be extremely safe. It also offers infinite variables for conditioning your body at every level of fitness, from beginner to elite: Vary the terrain and the incline, and add in load by wearing weight in the form of weight vests or loaded backpacks (or children!). Loaded walking, described below, is a powerful tool in even an advanced athlete's kit.

The second layer is *mobility work*. This refers to exercises that, simply stated, help you find the flow in your body so that moving feels easy and free. Mobility work matters because it helps to release stiffness and restriction in the muscles and connective tissues and restore the natural full range of motion of your joints. Range of motion means the joint's ability to go from its "closed" to "open" position, like when your shoulders allow your arms to circle fully overhead and behind you, or when your hips let you lift your knee up and circle it fully out to the side. Without that ability, you get sore and pained easily, can find it hard to do basic movements, and can injure yourself. If you've ever done shoulder circles, hip swivels, and Upward Dog in yoga, you've already done some mobility work.

Walking offers benefits to mobility and could actually be considered the first mobility drill. But given how much we sit today, often frozen in one position and frequently under stress, walking alone is not enough to keep the body open and able to move in a fluid, comfortable way. If you are actively strength training, it's even more important to do some mobility work. Your body builds strength in your muscles ten times faster than in the connective tissues of tendons and ligaments. If these all-important tissues haven't been conditioned in advance, it's easy to get overexcited, throw heavy stuff around, and blow a shoulder or injure a knee in the gym. Mobility work, the way I see it, helps build up the connective tissues and preps you to stay safe and supported before you up the ante and go fast and hard. It also helps you counterbalance your strength building with enough flexibility that the tissues stay pliable and supple, not short and tight, helping you move gracefully and find freedom and joy in your physicality.

So what does it involve? Sequences of exercises like scapula shrugs (a push-up that has you move *upward* from the starting position to create space in the upper back), yogic moves like Downward Dog, animal-flow moves like Bear Crawl, and martial-arts moves like jiu jitsu's stand-to-base motion get combined into fun drills that truly service the joints and tissues while building stability across the body and a stronger core. For all these reasons, the pyramid's second layer is vital because it contributes to protecting, preserving, restoring, and enhancing your ease of movement — a quality that is quickly lost when you sit or stand statically all day for work, or that gets locked up after sports or hard workouts. It contributes to longevity, too, because mobility tends to decrease as we age, more so if you let your everyday activity level decline and lose muscle mass to boot. By regularly practicing mobility work, you'll be able to move well for longer. I'd wager that mixing up movements in this way — getting up and down off the floor, walking like a gorilla dragging its knuckles, or half-tipped over like a bear — also helps you think differently and more creatively. Kids show us all the time — playing with their whole body and mixing up the ways they move is part and parcel of imagining new games and inventing wild ideas.

Mobility also refers to something incredibly obvious: *Move more throughout the day!* Some experts say that when it comes to staying healthy, the "nonintentional" movement you do outside of the gym, just getting yourself from point A to B to C is most important of all. In fact, experts now say if you sit all day and strength train for an hour and then sit some more, you essentially negate the benefits of your workout because your tissues "remodel" themselves into stronger versions after the workout is finished. If you're sedentary and stuck in a frozen position, guess what new shape your body takes on? So, before even worrying about programing your hard workout, go back a step. Ask how you can be a movement opportunist today. *How can I walk more, stand up and stretch more, get up and down more, and move in all directions from morning through night?*

The third layer is *strength*. This refers to the capacity of the muscles, bones, and connective tissues to carry load. You develop it by putting stress on the tissues and challenging them to handle more than normal — aka adding resistance. We all have a certain level of strength by virtue of carrying ourselves around. But having *more* of it leads to greater quality of life. Think of this as stepping up a level in health: You live longer, but now you do it with higher well-being and fewer complications. You become a stronger, more resilient person across the board. When you build more muscle, you increase your metabolism and feel more energized, especially as you age. You increase bone density, which helps protect your freedom to move actively as you age. You also protect and boost your brain function because physical challenge, especially intense demands like weight lifting, stimulates the release of proteins called neurotrophins that are important for the growth, health, and survival of certain brain cells. You also guard against pain — having stronger glute muscles, for example, will reduce chances of back pain, which is often a result of weakened glutes not holding the spine securely. You also start to change your body composition as muscles develop — if you've been wanting to see more shape, carve away fat, or put on a bit of mass, strength is where it's at. This also adds to quality of life not only because you start to enjoy the way you look and feel, but also because strength training tends to help bring on deep sleep, which your muscles require to do their nighttime repair.

You can develop strength in so many ways. Many of the mobility drills that follow, as well as the bodyweight exercises in the workouts like squats, planks, push-ups, and pull-ups will help you develop strength. Other bodyweight exercises that help to build strength include exercises like Pilates and yoga. Learning how to lift and move weight safely, whether through kettlebell or barbell training, free weights, supervised circuit training, or with a trainer at a gym mixing free weights and machines will develop strength further. All these things are excellent progressions from the basic workouts that follow.

The apex of the pyramid is *power.* This

is what you get when you combine strength with speed. Power helps you move quickly and forcefully, and I like to develop this by doing short, higher-intensity workouts. If you build power on top of the previous layers of walking, mobility, and strength, you can arrive at what I call a state of *higher performance*. Your body starts to show you what it's made of. It's like discovering you have a fifth gear you didn't know about. It's the quality that helps you transfer fitness off the mat or out of the gym and enables you to jump into new activities — like pickup basketball on the weekend — with gusto. It also transfers to endurance activities like running, biking, and swimming; it makes them easier.

The health benefits are multiple. By doing bursts of activity at a speed that forces you to work really hard, you train anaerobically — that's just a fancy term for working so hard your cells' demand for oxygen exceeds the oxygen available, and you start burning the fuel from food that's stored in your muscles and your liver, generating an overall greater fat-burning effect. (To simplify greatly, "aerobic" exercises such as low- to medium-intensity running or biking keeps your heart rate at a level where you primarily burn oxygen and carbohydrates;

As a beginner it's ideal to use body weight. This isn't lightweight stuff! It's more than possible to get ripped training only with your body weight. As you progress, however, you might want some variety. Consider training with dumbbells, kettlebells, barbells, or machines, if you choose. It doesn't stop there; once you have a baseline of stable strength, you want to up the challenge, testing the body to move odd things at odd angles while maintaining great form! This includes lifting things like Strongman stones, sandbags, and heavy medicine balls. Grappling with ungainly objects forces you to tighten up your core and brace yourself well. The benefits translate not just to well-rounded strength but also safe supported movements for all the unexpected demands of real life.

higher-intensity exercise bumps you into a new zone where you burn more of the fat stored in your body.) Burning body fat in this way is superefficient: a short workout can lead to up to forty-eight hours of your metabolism working hard; meanwhile the strength aspect of the workouts helps you build muscle. Now your body can really start to change shape! Though you can't see it, you help your blood-sugar-controlling hormone, insulin, work efficiently to keep your blood sugar in check, which massively reduces the risk of disease. And did I mention these power workouts make you sweat hard? That's essential for helping your body get out the waste and toxins that can accumulate when you're sedentary for too long.

One last thing: When you train for power, you get to express your inner animal in a healthy way — you liberate the part of you that feels bold but is told most of the time to sit down and keep quiet. When you push the edges of what you can do, explore the realm of discomfort, and complete something that asks for effort, you get to unleash your inner greatness — who wouldn't feel good doing that?

Power sits at the top of the pyramid because you don't want to leap into this kind of high-intensity training straight off the bat if you've been inactive. Getting your walking and mobility down for a few weeks is wise, then you can experiment with the beginner workouts that follow at a moderate pace, before upping the intensity.

A couple of more things about this pyramid

The Pyramid takes a while to build but is designed to last. This is neither a magic bullet "get shredded for a movie role in eight weeks" nor a "beach body overnight" approach to fitness. There's a difference between training for pure aesthetics versus building functional strength and fitness for life. What you may not realize is that the slow-and-steady route, done systematically, can get you to a similar place aesthetically — it just takes longer! So think of this as a one- to two-year mission to improve your body (or longer if you're seeking to revolutionize your physique). The benefit of slow and steady is that it gives you an unbreakable foundation of conditioning and resilience. Here's a secret from trainers who know this stuff: If you just train for aesthetics, working all day to torch fat and carve a new physique, sure you can look great. But the foundation is weaker: miss a few days and you begin to decondition. It also involves being absolutely fastidious with diet and super hard core about training. The slower path is more sustainable — you can miss some days, but you won't suffer for it.

of health and well-being: It's strongest when you give yourself dedicated time each week to play, freely and with no goal but to have physically uninhibited fun and explore what piques your curiosity, ideally with others — kids, pets, or friends — and when you also have plenty of time and space for active recovery so that gains made in the body get a chance to integrate and solidify. Fitness improvements actually occur after the workout.

Think of play and recovery as two watering holes next to the pyramid — places that restore you with cool water after all the sweaty effort to build, build, build.

And the ground this pyramid is standing on? It's more than it seems. There are two seriously impactful elements at the base of a well-constructed fitness pyramid, and we can't afford to overlook them if we want to see improvements in longevity, strength, and performance. These are good food and great sleep. No matter how gung-ho you are about your training, without nutrition and sleep in place, you're robbing your body of what it needs to really show you what it's made of. These elements are especially important if you want to see changes in weight and body composition, either by losing weight or gaining muscle mass.

Before we look at how we can translate

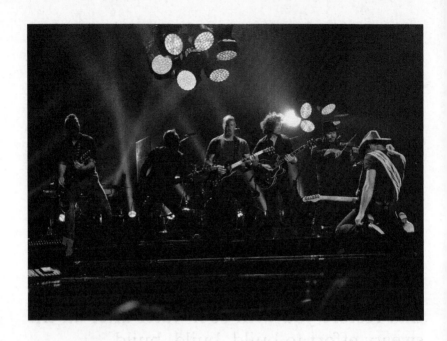

this pyramid into a formula, let's zoom in on the bricks from which it's made. These are the five foundational ideas that underlie this functional and integrated way of moving and training.

THE 4 PRINCIPLES OF FUNCTION

1 TRAIN YOUR BODY AS A WHOLE. Everything is connected; sounds obvious, but we often isolate parts of body in training or get stuck using muscles in the same planes of movement. Doing this increases the odds of injury, makes it harder to build a strong core, and is metabolically inefficient. Primal moves

like medicine ball slams and sledge-hammer chops ensure you use your full body to generate force in multidimensional ways — moving forward, side to side, and rotationally, which is key for generating power and building muscle mass.

2 **MOVE WELL, THEN GET STRONG.** You'll generate much less wear and tear if you learn how to do the basic "functional patterns" of natural human movement — squatting, crawling, walking, and running, lifting your arms overhead, and so forth — using the right muscles in the right ways. The mobility drills later in this chapter will help you enjoy your workouts now, as well as prevent problems down the line. Working with a well-qualified trainer is ideal for mastering basic moves if you can swing it, but, if not, you can also learn a lot from videos online.

3 **QUALITY OVER QUANTITY.** Balance moderation in duration and frequency with intensity of output. Keep length and frequency of workouts reasonable (the workouts that follow keep work output to about twenty minutes) in order to avoid overtraining, which can spike cortisol and trigger inflammation. Within the workout, however, remember bursts of intensity and even discomfort are part of your growth. It's a Goldilocks thing: find your sweet spot between "so hard you lose good form" and "so easy you're cruising." A workout should make you feel good, sometimes worked, but not wrecked!

4 PROGRESSION, PROGRESSION, PROGRESSION. The law of incremental adaptation means your body will adapt to challenge and figure out ways to make it easier, so if you want to keep growing in strength, speed, overall fitness — or simply in muscle definition — you have to keep upping the ante. That's why running the same three miles a day won't give you much gain over time. Once you've got your good form down, keep adding challenge to your workouts by mixing things up and changing the variables: perform them faster, add weight, or increase the complexity of movements.

Now that the basics are covered, let's put everything together into an action plan!

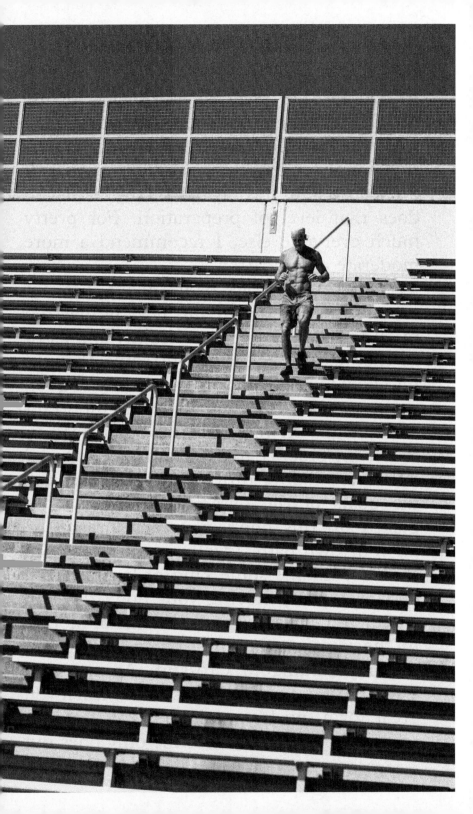

GETTING AFTER IT: YOUR PHYSICAL PRACTICE

In chapter 4, I gave you a preview of my typical training day when I'm on tour. I know — it's full on and can add up to several hours per day of physical exertion. Full disclosure: I'm the only one on my team who does that level of preparation. For pretty much everyone else, I recommend a more moderate approach.

As the quarterback of my team, I'm not exactly the coach, but I'm heavily invested in all the players being as healthy and as fit as they can be. So I've put some thought into how to get from somewhere shy of good shape to closer to your goal. It's important to say right off the bat: You don't need to follow my practice to get healthy and strong! There are lots of different ways to achieve the goals of the pyramid, and, if you've picked up this book, you may already be on your own path. Ideally, a good program should combine some kind of load bearing and resistance; moving your body through space; and expressing a full range of motion in the joints — anything from boot camp to bodybuilding to CrossFit. At our gym TRUMAV, we created classes that teach you great form, push your limits, and test you mentally — but we're not the only ones out there. If you've found something you love that is helping you develop and progress — by all means, stick with it!

If you haven't started any of that yet, don't worry. Use the following practices to build your own pyramid — then you'll be in great shape for whatever form of fitness calls your name down the line. What I've discovered from helping a whole crew of people get healthy is that you build momentum when you come out of the gate strong and have some easy wins at the start. You don't have to be a badass from the get-go; it's smarter to work back up to where you used to be — college athlete, buff young Turk back in the day — by giving your body the time and space to incrementally make gains. You'll find a progression here with all four layers of the pyramid put into action. Walking and mobility are two separate practices you can do daily or on alternate days while strength is developed by doing the power workouts.

With that said, here's some advice for tailoring the program to your fitness level:

BEGINNER: If you feel out of shape, focus on walking and doing mobility drills. Your week will look like this: Alternate a walk and mobility practice five days per week. (If you have time to do both on one day, do them both!) One day a week: If you have the capacity, do one long walk (three to five miles). If that's out of reach, work up to that goal in stages over time — one mile, two miles, and so on. One day a week: Take a play day, as described on page 381–386. Do this for two to three weeks, then pick a workout and just do one round of it and see how it feels. Do it at 50 percent capacity — take it easy. Every three days, try another workout in the same low-key fashion, slowly getting familiar with this way of moving until you feel you can up the intensity. (Use a mobility drill as a warm-up each time.)

INTERMEDIATE: If you are already active but haven't done much functional fitness training, do a thirty-minute walk five times a week, and two to three times a week do the workouts marked beginner, aiming for three times a week, always doing a mobility drill as your warm-up. All total, this will add up to an hour a day. On the days when you don't have time for this, prioritize walking and mobility. If you have time for a long walk (five miles plus) once per week, go for it. At least once a week, try to get in some kind of purely play-based activity — with all that good training going on, you deserve to have some fun!

ADVANCED: If you are already proficient in this style of training, walk daily and three to four times a week do any of the workouts, either intermediate or advanced depending on your fitness level, with a mobility drill as your warm-up. On the days you don't have time for all of this, prioritize walking and mobility. If you find time for one long walk (five miles plus), that's extra credit. Be sure to remember to play at least once a week, too.

THE SMALLEST STEP

No matter what level you are starting from, I encourage you to experiment with including one, two, or all three steps of the "clearing" exercise (page 155–157) before you start moving. These steps can even *be* your workout if you're struggling to start for any reason. Breathing and releasing are two important kinds of movement in and of themselves that get energy moving through your body in subtle but powerful ways. You have plenty of time to get strong and fit! The key is to do something for your body consistently, not missing more than a day or two. If active breathing is your "workout" for now, do it with gusto! Trust that it's the start of your new lifestyle.

If you are an experienced athlete who is working out hard three times a week or more, be sure to include some recovery activities if you can; they're the treat for your tissues that helps gains really get ingrained. I don't suggest the everyday athlete do hard workouts five times a week; that puts you at risk for overtraining.

This is not a rigid program; there will be times when you might only be able to do one thing a day. In those cases, get your walk in first and foremost. Load it with weight if you want some extra challenge.

LEVEL 1: WALKING

I love starting my morning with a walk to get my body loose and alert first thing in the day. I'm lucky to have the luxury of a full hour to do this, but even twenty to thirty minutes if time's tight will have huge benefit. Though much of my walking happens on a treadmill, partly because I travel a lot, the best kind of walking is outside in nature, especially if you can vary your terrain on different days. That said — use what you've got! On my treadmill, I walk at a brisk pace but keep it (flat) for the first half of my walk, then start dialing up the incline every five minutes.

Making a daily walk your first fitness goal

is a powerful act. It is easy to do, requires minimal equipment, and can be done solo or with a companion — human or animal. It should also be an *ongoing* fitness goal during your whole athletic journey because even when you're an advanced athlete, it can be your warm-up, your recovery, and, if needed, your rehab. You might start with ten minutes; that's okay. But have a target to work toward of at least thirty minutes once a day minimum at a pace that feels natural to you (not all the benefits of walking are cardiovascular, so if you don't feel the urge or the ability to walk briskly, that's totally fine. You don't have to "learn" how to walk, but sometimes it's good to remember a natural, easy walking style. It starts by leaving all devices at the door and finding your feet. Yes, you know where your feet are, but do you ever stop to feel how the soles of your feet connect to the ground? Wearing walking shoes that are as close to barefoot as possible — really thin in the sole — will help here, and whenever possible, like on the beach, walk barefoot! You actually get extra benefits from closer contact with the ground — recent research shows that the pressure of your foot against the earth increases blood circulation in the brain, optimizing your brain function and overall sense of well-being.

Take a minute to wiggle your feet and feel every part of them ground into the earth; your feet are built with an extraordinary amount of muscles we never even notice and you want to wake them all up, plus the receptors that help activate the muscles in the legs. Now start walking. Hands swinging freely at your sides, and feeling the ground underfoot with each step, breathe in through your nose letting your belly softly inflate and deflate. (Extra credit: Tongue resting gently on the roof of your mouth helps this breath happen naturally.) Imagine the breath expanding your spine upward so your posture pulls up and you stand tall. Relax your face, take in your surroundings, and enjoy!

One of the best ways to retrain your posture as well as build strength through walking is to add load or some other kind of stimulus. Don't do this on every walk; but if you'd like to try it, do it every third or fourth walk. The safest way to add weight is with a weight vest (weighted with up to 10 percent of your body weight) because it distributes the weight equally on your front and back. These don't have to cost a fortune, and they can be a great tool in your kit. Weight vests evenly distribute load from all directions and compress the trunk, which gives

Sometimes it's good to turn your walk into something that's a little more down and dirty. Especially if the only chance you have to exercise is your daily walk. Rest assured there are infinite ways to add mobility and strength building exercises to Fido's morning stroll or your forty minutes with your walking group! Here's how.

- Before setting off, take a few moments to do a few simple hip circles, shoulder circles, arm circles and any other shoulder mobility exercises you know. Add in a few Mobility Drill exercises, yoga stretches, or animal flow movements.
- During your walk, every five minutes add in reps of exercises from the workout section. You could start by doing rounds of five reps each of basic body weight moves: five Squats, five Lunges, five Push-ups (try these on your knees if you are just starting out). Every third or fourth walk, try this wearing your weight vest for extra challenge!
- Once you're in the groove, diversify this formula. Every few minutes

(between three and five) do five to ten reps of other movements such as High Knees, Planks, Broad Jumps, or Burpees; use a park bench to do dips or steps, or a high bar in a playground to do pull-ups or negative pull-ups (where you jump up then very slowly lower down to build pull-up capacity). Why not add some sprints or relay back and forth between points with your friends! You can certainly extend your walk to longer than thirty minutes if you'd like; no matter how much time you have, you'll get a great workout in by adding these strength and plyometric moves. In terms of how many exercises and reps to do, feel into your capacity and the intensity you want — if your form is getting sloppy it's a sign you're doing too much. (I don't recommend wearing a weight vest if you are doing explosive moves like burpees and broad jumps.)

you stability as you move while causing you to reflexively improve your posture. (If you don't have one, two backpacks on the front and back — try filling them with bags of sand.) Loaded walks add challenge, which you want to get healthier! Another great training option for finding good posture and building good movement is *removing load* by walking in water! Try walking back and forth across the shallow end of the pool — it's more challenging than it seems. (If you want to develop A-game walking form that's maximally efficient and connects your breath to your motions, check out a method called Chi Walking, which you can learn about online.)

As you get comfortable walking, try to build variety of terrain into your walks. Find routes that involve hills and let them help add challenge: incline and speed are two ways to dial up intensity. Also, think about different surfaces you can walk on — grass, dirt, sand, snow, gravel — that change the inputs to your body, adding variation and new stimuli.

Once a week, aim to do a long walk of close to five miles; these longer walks serve an important purpose. Not only do they let you get out into new terrain and see new sights, but they also toughen all the connective tissues in your body and build endurance as postural muscles work extra hard.

How to Walk Well

- Plan a route that you feel safe doing, and bring a friend or companion if you're not sure about walking solo.
- Make it a group activity. Walking, as my sister Sandy discovered, is the absolute easiest way to meet up with like-minded people. Put the word out, show up where you say you will, and watch your walking club grow.
- Check the weather before you go and take adequate layers, a bottle of water if it's going to be a hot day, and safety strips or a headlamp if it will be foggy or dark.
- Stack it. Stacking means merging a few things together so that your walking time serves other purposes if you're short of time. This is intentional — it's not the same thing as getting distracted and checking out. It just means your walk doesn't have to be a totally purist exercise experience each and every time. Maybe it gets you to work and back or takes you on all your errands. Or it's your time for connecting with a buddy instead of meeting for coffee; or you have "walking meetings" with colleagues (it might inspire creativity). Maybe it's your time for listening to a

podcast, an audiobook, or a coaching call. If you have a dog, chances are, it's when you walk him. If your mind says, "I don't have time to walk!" ask, "What can I stack onto this exercise session?"

- It's great to get outside in all kinds of weather if you have the shoes and clothes for it. Assuming you can stay warm and dry, practice getting out in all kinds of climates. If the weather really doesn't cooperate, do a mobility drill instead.

- Whenever possible, go green. Studies show walking in natural environments rather than urban ones helps your mind stop worrying and reduces negative thinking. It's also extremely beneficial to kids' states of mind. "Green outdoor activity" is also shown to reduce symptoms of ADHD significantly.

- After your walk, take a moment to ask yourself the 8 questions on page 170–171. It only takes a minute, and it's important to notice the small shifts here and there that reinforce your healthy habits. It's amazing how something as simple as walking can make a huge difference in the way you feel!

Progressing to Running

Is running the natural progression after you've been walking for a while? Not necessarily! In fact, as a blanket statement it's better and safer to stick to walking, just adding challenges as discussed above. This is especially true if you're overweight; you want to condition your joints, not stress them through running. But if running is something you love doing, there's plenty to enjoy. Consider taking the time to build strength and mobility through the workouts here for several weeks *before* launching into running. Then start with fast, steep uphill runs: try an interval of twenty seconds' effort followed by three minutes rest/off, and repeat. This helps build the solid base of strength for longer runs later. As a general rule, if you do work up to running, keep your runs to about thirty minutes and combine with the workouts here. Because of the wear and tear on the body that running creates, it's wise to keep regular running as part of a rotation — do regular runs for only one month out of three or four — so you don't create too much tissue breakdown. Rest assured if you are doing smart full-body training workouts, you will be in great condition for whatever race or running challenge you want to pursue, even with this rotation schedule.

LEVEL 2: MOBILITY

Your mobility drills serve two purposes. On their own, they are a short, functional practice designed to preserve, restore, and enhance your body's ability to move well, safely, and without restriction. They also serve as your warm-ups before the workouts that follow because they get your circulation going and get all your body parts moving up to speed — think loose and stable at once — before you start adding challenge through speed and strength. I know the term *warm-up* typically makes you think of doing things like jumping jacks and jump roping. Those kinds of things are great, too — but if you've not been active for a while, mobility drills are much kinder on your joints, and, even for experienced athletes, they give you a chance to practice new movements for a few minutes as you warm up. They also are phenomenal for checking into your body, exploring where tension is being held, and then moving that tension out. They let you reverse some of the negative effects of sitting too long or simply spending hours under stress — which also makes them great routines for days you're in a slump or don't have the mojo to get to a full workout. If you're like me, over time, you'll see them as a treat for your whole system, not a chore. Once Roger helped me see the value in these drills, I haven't looked back.

The following mobility drills are designed to increase your range of motion, build and restructure connective tissues, and develop the ability to hold your core tight for stability and grace. They each consist of five rounds of three to six movements that are repeated a specific number of time sequences. You don't need a yoga mat or any special equipment to do them.

The drills are designed to be used as follows for maximum benefit: Follow one drill for four to six weeks, then try the next. This helps you stick with certain movements long enough to functionally build capacity in the areas of the body that are being addressed, helping to strengthen the connective tissue over time. This gradual build is more effective than jumping between different exercises day to day. Think of it almost like "remodeling" your house; when you take time to work on one room until it's refurbished, then move to the next, you really begin to see improvement coming together. Perform these at a speed that lets you be precise, but not so slow they feel easy. After you're familiar with a drill, it should take about fifteen minutes to perform.

There is a plethora of mobility moves you

can start to learn when you have these basics down. In our workouts we love to include other fun animal moves like Gorilla Walks and Chimp Walks. If you prefer more guidance, another option is one of Roger's favorite resources, the Functional Patterns 10-Week Online Training Course, created by movement maverick Naudi Aguilar. This course is especially good if you're experiencing restriction or pain; it helps you release the tension compromising your movements and teaches you all about developing good movement patterns.

DRILL #1 / FIVE ROUNDS

1. Bear Crawl 10 steps
2. Infinity Drill x 10
3. Mountain Climber x 20
4. Deep Squat, hold for 30 seconds
5. V-Sit Leg Raise x 10
6. Box Hop Hold x 10

BEAR CRAWL Start on all fours with your hands directly under your shoulders and your knees under your hips. Press your hips up to come onto your toes with your knees raised off the ground several inches, and your arms straight. Keeping your core tight and your back flat, travel forward with your

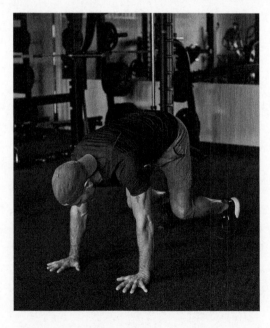

right hand and left foot moving in tandem and landing together, and then your left hand and right foot. Count one step each time your left hand hits the ground.

INFINITY DRILL Start in Bear Crawl position (page 318) with your hands under your shoulders and your knees slightly bent. Sweep your right leg behind you as if trying to kick someone standing on your left. As your body turns to follow it, your left foot will pivot onto its outside edge, your left leg will become straight, and your right hand will come off the ground. Land your right foot flat on the ground as close to your left hand as possible, with your shin vertical and your right hand, floating near your face.

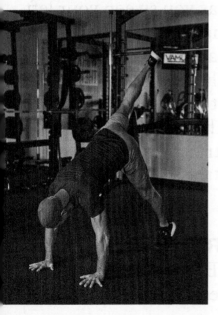 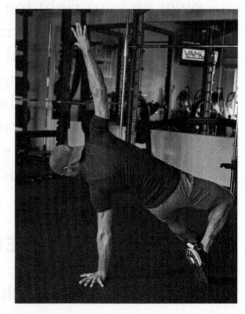

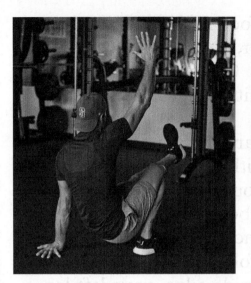
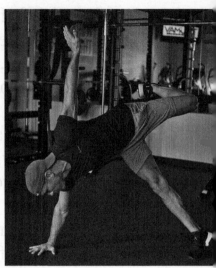

That's the first half of the loop.

Now pick your left ankle, knee, and hip off the ground and draw your left foot close to your body, then thread it between the hand and foot that are still on the ground. Start to pivot on your right toe as you sweep your left leg behind you, "kicking" an imaginary person on your right, and as your body opens to the sky, place your right hand on the floor. Land your left foot flat on the ground close to your right hand, with your left shin vertical as your right leg straightens. Each time a foot sweeps and taps the ground counts as one rep.

MOUNTAIN CLIMBER Start in plank position with a tight core. Bring your right knee forward under your chest and land your toes

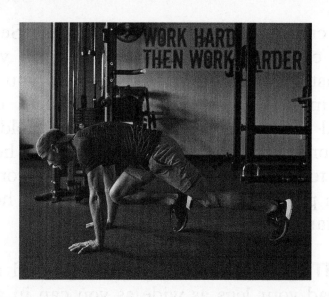

on the ground. Now swap your feet: Return your right foot to plank position as you bring your left knee and foot forward. That is one rep. Pick up a quick pace, almost as if you are "climbing" in a plank position.

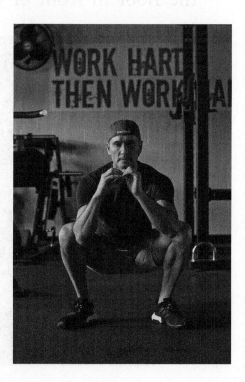

DEEP SQUAT Stand with your heels under your hips and your feet turned outward to 30 degrees. Press all four corners of your feet into the ground to distribute weight evenly. Lower your butt until your hip crease is lower than your knee. See if you can take the squat deeper until your hamstrings are on your calves and you are "sitting." You may press your knees outward with your elbows to balance. Hold on to something in front of you if this helps you to sink deeper. Hold for thirty seconds, then push the ground away with your heels to stand.

V-SIT LEG RAISE Sit on the ground and spread your legs as wide as you can in a V, engaging your core and sitting up as straight as possible, and placing your hands on the floor in front of you or behind you for

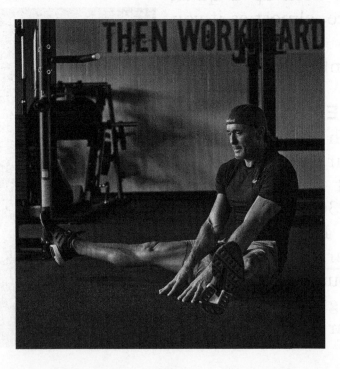

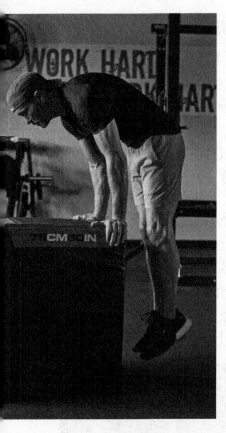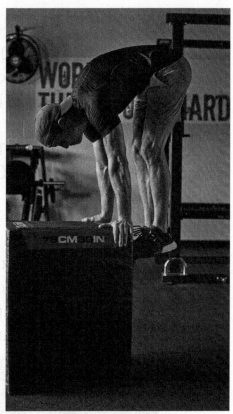

balance. Point your toes, raise your legs as high as you can, and lower.

BOX HOP HOLD Place your hands flat on plyometric box turned on it longest side or on a countertop. Pressing with your hands, jump up as if you are trying to make your feet level with the box, land quickly, and jump again. Get your hips as high as you can — but not so high you lose control. You should feel a slight "pause" at the very top of the movement.

DRILL #2 / FIVE ROUNDS

1. Stand to Base x 10 total (5 each side)
2. Rolling Candlestick x 10
3. Rolling Backbend Prep x 10 total (5 each side)
4. Oil Pump Squat x 10
5. Scapula Shrug x 10

STAND TO BASE Stand with your feet wider than hip-width apart. Bend down and place your right hand about four inches in front of your right foot. Pick your right foot up and slide it through the right hand and the left foot, slightly above the ground, with

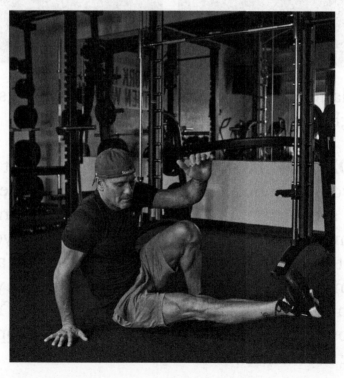

your right butt cheek touching the ground when you get to full extension. Now reverse it: Pick up your right foot, knee, and hip off the ground first, then draw your foot back through to its starting position, flat on the floor by your hand, and stand up. Now do the same with the left leg.

ROLLING CANDLESTICK Start lying on the floor with your legs extended and arms by your side. Roll your shoulders, reaching your feet to the sky, extending your legs fully at the top of the movement, then roll back down. Your hands may touch the floor until you can do this with your hands in front of

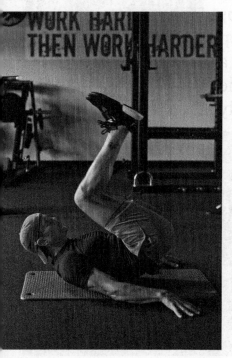
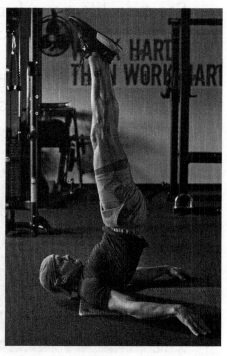

your chest. Do not roll onto your neck or into a yoga plough pose.

To modify, start by simply hugging your knees and rolling onto your shoulders; then start to raise your feet into the air on each roll, and finally come into a full candlestick.

ROLLING BACK-BEND PREP Come into a squat and place your right hand on the ground behind your right shoulder and slightly out to the side. Start to lift your hips to the sky and sweep your left hand in a giant circle over the right side of your body

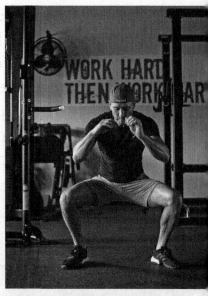

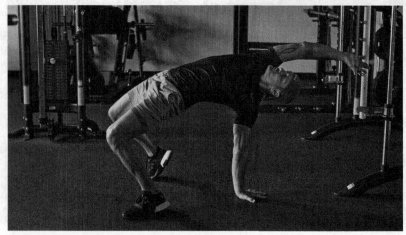

and toward the back, left corner of the room as your chest and hips open to the sky. Reverse the motion to come back to a squat. Switch sides.

OIL PUMP SQUAT Start in a tabletop position with your hands and knees on the ground. Bring your hands in close to your knees, about one hand's length away, and raise your knees one inch off the ground. Pump your hips up to the sky then come back down to starting position.

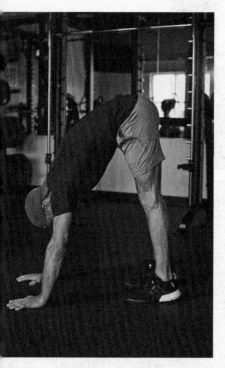
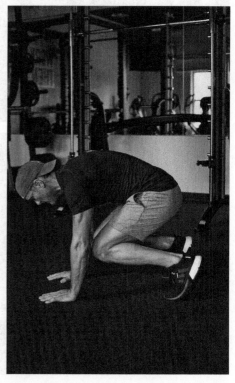

SCAPULA SHRUG Stand with your arms extended in front of you. Keeping your entire body tight, pull your shoulder blades together tightly enough to crush a pencil, then release and round your shoulder blades as far as you can to create a dome. Remember to keep your chin and head neutral. Don't jut your neck in and out. Move from your back and shoulders only.

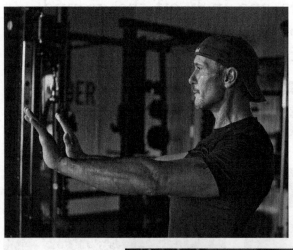

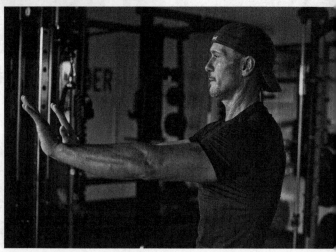

DRILL # 3 / FIVE ROUNDS

1. Lie Down Stand Up x 10
2. Stiff Leg Hop x 10
3. Lateral Squat Push-up x 10 (5 each side)
4. Hip Hike Walk (forward and backward) x 10 steps each direction
5. Elevated Cobra 90 seconds

LIE DOWN STAND UP This is as simple as it sounds. Start by lying down on your back and get back up to a standing position in any way except by crossing your feet. You can squat and bring one hand to the floor

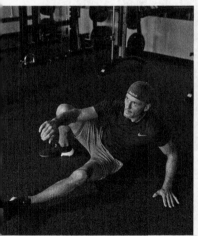
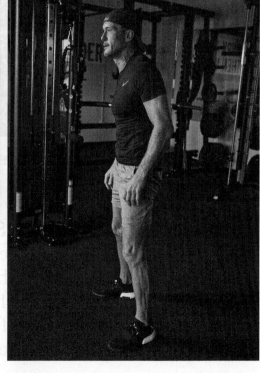

or even get onto your knees first for added assistance. Then bring yourself to standing any way you want *without crossing your feet*. If you put your right hand to the floor as support on the first rep, use your left hand on the second.

STIFF LEG HOP
Stand with your feet, ankles, and knees together. Lock your legs, squeeze your glutes and thighs super tight, and tighten your core. Make small hops forward *without bending your knees* but keeping toes, heels, and knees together. You will look a little like 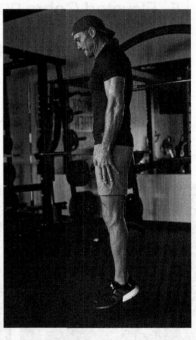 a pogo stick. Don't worry about how far or high you hop.

LATERAL SQUAT PUSH-UP Start in a deep squat with your heels on the ground. Tip 90 degrees over to the right side of your body, placing your right hand on the ground diagonally behind you, far enough out that your elbow does not touch your body as

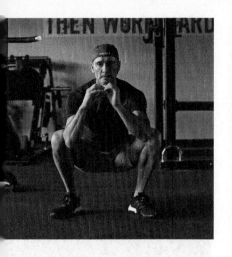

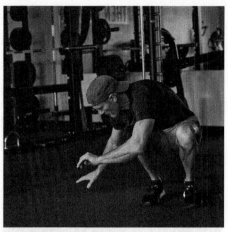

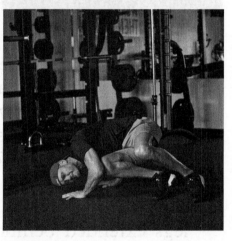

you lower, then place your left hand down about twelve inches to the left. Looking down, tip until your right ear and right knee touches the ground — your heels will likely come off the ground here — then press back up. Now tip to the left side.

HIP HIKE WALK Start seated on the ground with your legs extended straight in front of you and your hands clasped at your chest. Lift your right heel, knee, hip, and butt cheek off the ground *without bending*. Now reach your leg forward a few inches, then place your butt down. That is one step. Now lift your left leg in the same way, reach

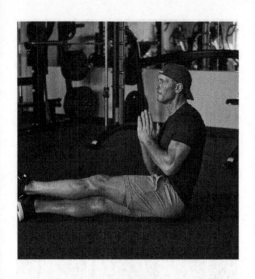
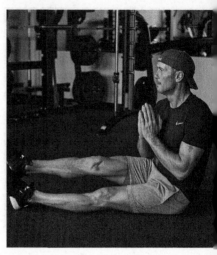

forward a few inches without bending it, and set your left butt cheek down. Continue for ten "steps" forward and ten "steps" back.

This exercise helps maintain the all-important ability to lift your hip, something that degenerates with sedentary life and age.

ELEVATED COBRA Lie facedown with your legs extended behind you in a relaxed position. Place your hands on a low box or bench, ladder rung, or coffee table (or a Stahl bar at the gym) with your hands facing palm down. Scoot your hips back a few inches until

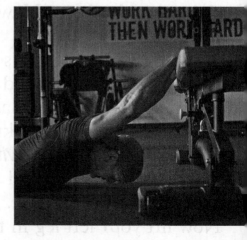

your arms are fully extended and lock your elbows. Press your chest to the ground by driving your armpits downward. There is no other movement. This is just a stretch.

LEVELS 3–4: STRENGTH & POWER

If you were to spy on my band and me training, you'd see lots of oscillating battle ropes, upside-down people doing handstand push-ups against a wall, and others doing drills up and down stadium steps. We alternate faster drills on some days that really elevate our heart rates with slightly slower workouts on other days where weights get a little heavier and the workout's more of a grind. If you were getting technical, you might call this hybrid style of workout SHIFFT, for Short High(ish) Intensity Functional Fitness Training. They're hybrid because they fuse all kinds of movements together using body weight some of the time and added weight other times. This helps to target the metabolic conditioning aspect, strength building, and putting the body through its full range of motion — a three-in-one winning combo.

To help you experience these benefits, I've adapted my workouts into fairly simple variations that will achieve similar effects. There is minimal equipment required: You can do almost all the beginner variations with only your body. (Rest assured that using your body weight only is extremely effective; it sets you up for good stability and builds a foundation of strength so that you can add load later.) Intermediate and advanced variations are where you build power. You can use jump ropes and dumbbells to increase the intensity, and if you have access to a gym, you'll have the option to use equipment like rowers, bikes, and battle ropes as well.

Don't fall into the trap of thinking these workouts look too basic. They are designed to develop strength and power while keeping the movement pretty simple. They're short but impactful. If you're used to doing long runs, bike rides, or other cardio activity as your primary form of exercise, know that these workouts achieve efficient cardio conditioning in short time without the catabolic (breaking down) effect of endurance training that, if done to excess, can be stressful on the system.

If you've dipped your toe into high-intensity training of any kind, like interval training or Tabata drills (a drill programmed around eight rounds of twenty seconds on, ten seconds off), you may have heard the umbrella term *metabolic conditioning*. These strength and power workouts fit into this category — they require working hard in bursts of effort to train and condition your metabolism to work efficiently. Technically, you can engage in different levels of metabolic conditioning, working at different levels of intensity to train the body's three power output systems. But let's keep it simple for now. Work at the highest intensity you can get while *still maintaining good form.* If you are maintaining absolute perfect form during each rep with relative ease (performing like a straight-A student), then work a little harder. You want to hit a solid B average, which can be up to 15 to 20 percent shy of perfect form; the idea is to work at an intensity that feels challenging and gets you breathing hard, but is not impossible (and most definitely not painful). You should be really getting after it! If your form veers toward a C grade, meaning it's getting wiggly or messy, slow down the pace and correct it — or even stop and reset it, as it can lead to injury. In some of the workouts, you'll be directed to take a four-minute rest after multiple rounds of work or after a sprint session. This break seems long, but it has a purpose: it resets the energy system and is fundamental to accessing the stored fuel in your reserves. The break *helps* you to recruit energy to power through the latter rounds — so don't speed past it.

The eleven workouts that follow each have

a beginner, intermediate, and advanced variation. Choose the level that feels right for your ability, and if it's too easy, scale up; if it's too hard, scale down. (Several advanced workouts use significantly heavy weights and are intended for those with experience; read carefully before choosing your level.) You will want to have a timer on hand for many of them. Some intermediate and advanced variations use a jump rope. Where a box is called for (a "plyometric box" used in many gyms) you can substitute furniture or other options — you won't be jumping onto it. Where bike sprints are offered, try to use a fan bike if possible. These bikes don't need to be set to a certain resistance; they respond to the intensity of your effort. If you don't have access to one, set the bike tension to a level that will have you working very close to your maximum effort — fast and hard! Rowing machines are a terrific alternative.

Where instructed to do "as many rounds as possible" in a set number of minutes (otherwise known as AMRAP workouts), you are on your own to determine if and when you need to rest. The goal is to push it — so try to keep moving! Rest only if you truly need it.

Throughout the instructions you'll be

Short workouts that repeat several exercises quickly over multiple rounds seem super simple. Yet they will test you physically and test you mentally even more. Consider them a lesson in going deep. How do you give it your all as the clock keeps ticking? Here's a cheat sheet:

THE EARLY ROUNDS: You come out blazing with lots of momentum, but pace yourself! You don't want to burn out too quickly. You do want to establish good form and set the standard for the workout.

THE MIDDLE ROUNDS: These are about pure stamina. Keep up the effort and fall into a rhythm — not so overeager that you get sloppy, but not complacent. It should feel challenging!

THE FINAL ROUNDS: These are all about mental toughness. Push into your discomfort zone, know that you can finish strong. It's time to empty the tank! Give your best effort — it's not supposed to get easier, it's supposed to feel hard! If your form is getting a "C," modify the movement so it's easier (use the beginner or intermediate variation listed).

AFTER YOU CROSS THE FINISH LINE: Remember to celebrate! A few fist bumps and high fives are in order.

asked to "tighten your core." This is not the same as just pulling in your abs, and it's important to know the difference. Tightening your core involves a positive tension that creates a pillar of strength and safety. Your core is the entire central cylinder of your body from your pelvis all the way up to your chest, comprised of multiple muscles that keep you stable and solid, allowing you to gain whole-body strength while protecting your spine and preventing injury.

The exercise below will help you learn how to activate this cylindrical core so that you can develop the muscle memory to bring a tight core to all of your workouts. You should repeat this exercise frequently until you become very familiar with the feeling of a tight, engaged core.

BACK COMPRESSION CRUNCH Lie down on your back with your legs extended on the floor and your arms by your sides. Imagine you have an egg under your lower back. Inhale, then try to crush the egg through the force of compression, pushing your core cylinder outward and downward, *flattening your spine to the floor.* It's tricky, so play with it! Your abdomen should be flat, not curving into a C. Crush the egg, release. Repeat five times.

How to Work Out Well

If you are unfamiliar with using weights, it's a good idea to talk to a trainer about form before you get started. There are also a number of free resources online that teach correct form. Start with weights that challenge you slightly, and work your way up.

Start each workout with the mobility drill you've selected for this month. That will be your warm-up.

During your workout, work at the highest intensity and speed you can with good B-grade form.

Where instructions indicate to use 1/4, 1/3, or 1/2 body weight, this refers to the weight of the kettlebell or dumbbell you should use. Divide your body weight by 1/4, 1/3, or 1/2 and find the closest kettlebell or dumbbell to that weight. For example, if you weigh 150 pounds, 1/4 of your body weight is about 37 pounds. You might pick up a 35-pound kettlebell. If the suggested weight feels like too much to use safely and with good form, or if you are new to strength training, scale down as needed.

At the end of each workout, spend a few minutes of loose and lazy walking around to cool down. You don't need to do a dedicated "stretch" session, as you have been stretching your muscles during the workout (whether you realize it or not) and your frequent mobility sessions will keep you limber. These final moments are about breathing and feeling the energy you created moving through you.

Remember, even more important than anything you do in the five minutes after the workout is what you do in the rest of the day! Get up and move for a few minutes frequently in multiple directions to balance out the strength and power training. Your body will be best served if several times a day you drop into some squats and do a few Scapula Shrugs or Bear Crawls, or any other mobility-enhancing moves you already know. So what if your office mates think it's funny looking, or your kids decide you're a perfect vehicle to climb on? It will help make sure you get the *full gains* of your hard work, and move forward instead of backward in your strength, growth, and comfort.

STRENGTH AND POWER WORKOUTS

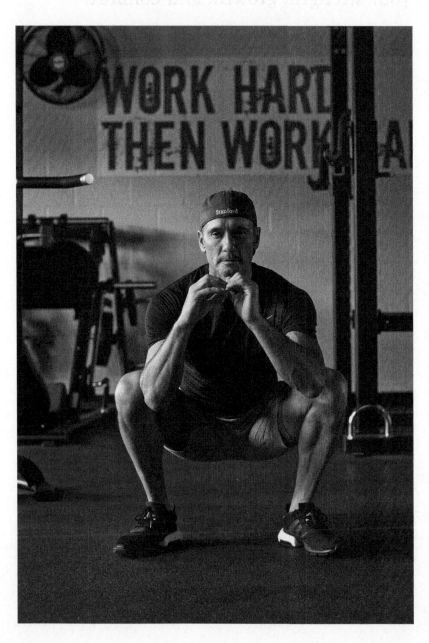

Fifteen-minute AMRAP workout. Do as many rounds as possible in fifteen minutes. One round is five push-ups, five squats.

Beginner	Intermediate	Advanced
Chest-Elevated Push-up x 5	Chest-to-Ground Push-up x 5	Feet-Elevated Push-up x 5
Squat x 5	Goblet Squat, 1/4 body weight x 5	Thruster, 1/4 body weight in each hand x 5

PUSH-UP

Beginner: Chest-Elevated Push-up. Place your hands on a box or countertop, hands slightly turned out and elbow creases facing forward. Walk your feet out to an inclined plank, making a straight line from shoulders to feet. Lower your chest to the box and push back to starting position keeping your

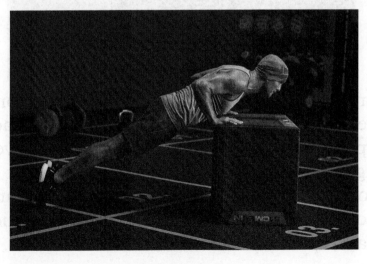

core and glutes tight. You can increase the difficulty when you're ready by using a box or bar that is lower to the floor. The closer to the floor, the harder it will be.

Intermediate: Chest-to-Ground Push-up. Start in a plank position with your hands directly under your shoulders and slightly turned out, your arms locked and elbow creases facing forward, your core tight, your heels above your toes. Maintain the plank position as you lower your body all the way

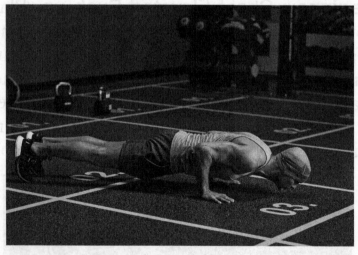

until your chest touches the ground. Don't lie down though! Immediately press back up by engaging your core and glutes even tighter and pushing out through your feet as you use your whole body to push up to plank position. (Imagine a cord pulling your mid-back upward.)

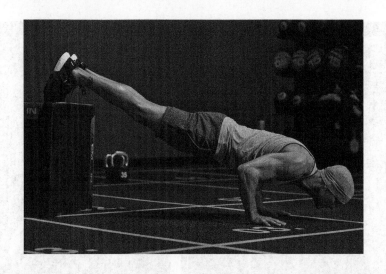

Advanced: Feet-Elevated Push-up. Do a full Chest-to-Ground Push-up with your feet elevated on a box, chair, TRX, or rings. Experiment with different heights and explore your range.

SQUAT

Beginner: Basic Squat. Stand with heels under your hips, feet a little wider than hip-width apart, and your toes pointed out to 30 degrees. Press the balls of your feet, your pinkie toes, and your heels into the ground to distribute your weight evenly. Lower your butt until your hip crease is lower than your knee. Push the ground away with your heels to stand. To scale this down, place a chair or box behind you and reach for it with your butt, sit briefly on it, then push back up to stand.

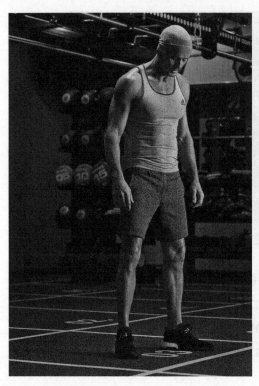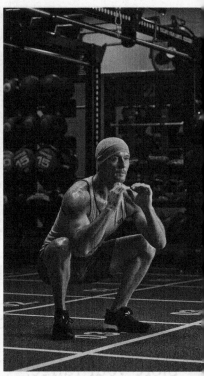

Intermediate: Goblet Squat. Hold a dumb-bell at one end so it is parallel to your spine, or a kettlebell by the horns. Keeping your shoulders back, elbows tight to your sides, and core tight, squat as above. Use a quarter of your body weight.

Advanced: Thruster. Hold one dumbbell at each shoulder, handles parallel. Squat and stand in one fluid motion, pushing the weights overhead with your palms facing forward or slightly rotated inwards, keeping your core tight. Use a quarter of your body weight in each hand.

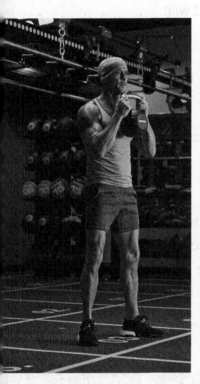
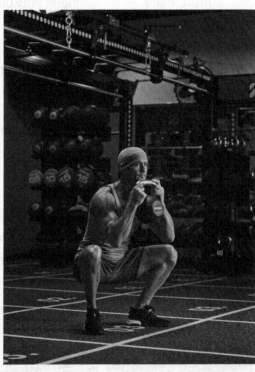

Do seven rounds of these three exercises.

Beginner	Intermediate	Advanced
Basic Plank Walkout x 5	Plank Walkout with Push-up x 5	Hindu Push-up x 5
Half Burpee (no push-up, no jump) x 10	Full Burpee x 10	Full Burpee Broad Jump x 10
Lazy Walk x 10 seconds	Stiff Leg Hops x 10	Stiff Leg Hops x 10

PLANK WALKOUT

Beginner: Basic. Stand with your feet under your hips. With bent or straight legs, place your palms on the ground. Walk out your hands until you are in a plank position. Walk your hands back to your feet and stand up.

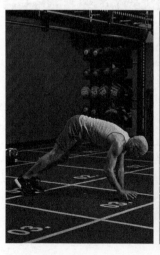
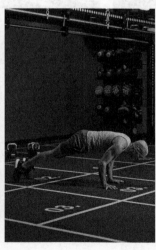
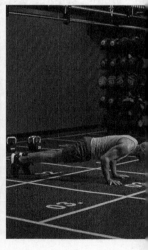

Intermediate: Do a **Plank Walkout**, adding a push-up in the plank position.

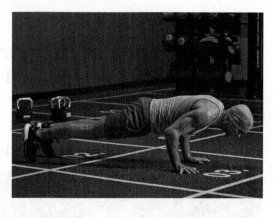

Advanced: Hindu **Push-up.** Start in Downward Dog, hips high and arms straight. Dive downward, then slide your nose, chest, and hips forward, a few inches above the ground. (Imagine sliding under barbed wire.) Rise into Upward Dog. Reverse the movement, sliding back under the wire and into Downward Dog. (If this is too hard, push back into Downward Dog.)

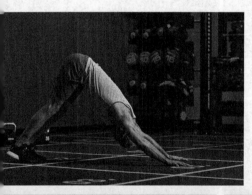

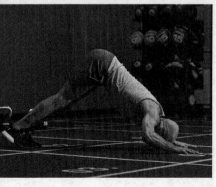

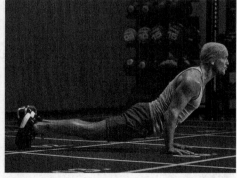

BURPEE

Beginner: Half Burpee. From standing, bend your knees and place your hands on the ground outside your feet. Hop your feet back to plank position, then hop them back outside your hands. Stand up.

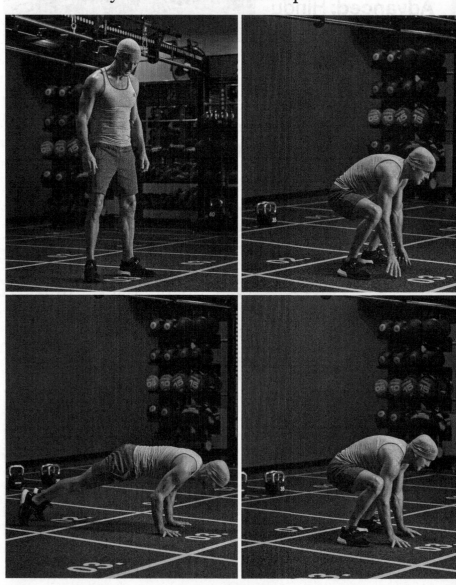

Intermediate: **Full Burpee.** When you get down to plank position, add one push-up. After you bring your feet outside your hands, add a jump and clap as you stand up.

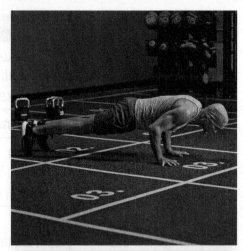

Advanced: **Full Burpee Broad Jump.** Do a Full Burpee and add a Broad Jump when you come up. Explode forward as far as you can, landing in a squat.

Lazy Walk: Walk slowly on a treadmill or back and forth in your workout space. Keep moving, but exert minimum effort.

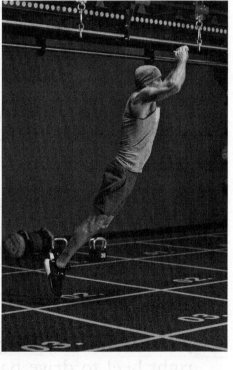

Stiff Leg Hops (see page 330).

Fifteen-minute AMRAP workout: Do as many rounds as possible of four exercises in fifteen minutes. Fan bikes are the preferred bikes for the bike sprint version.

Beginner	Intermediate	Advanced
Sprint for 30 seconds. You can run, bike, or row.	Sprint for 30 seconds. You can run, bike, or row.	Sprint for 30 seconds. You can run, bike, or row.
Lunge x 5 each side	Split Squat x 5 each side	Loaded Split Squat holding 1/4 body weight in each hand
Chest-Elevated Push-up x 15	Chest-to-Ground Push-up x 15	Feet-Elevated Push-up x 15
Jumping Jacks x 20	Jump Ropes x 40	Double Unders x 40

LUNGE

Beginner: Lunge. Stand with your feet hip-width apart and core tight. Take a big step forward with your right foot, keeping your upper body straight. Lower your body until your right thigh is parallel to floor and your right shin is vertical. You may lightly tap your left knee to the ground. Press into your right heel to drive back up to starting position, feet under hips.

Intermediate: Split Squat. Place a chair or box behind you. Ideally it will be the

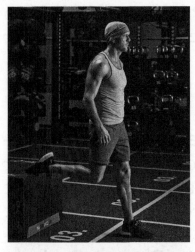
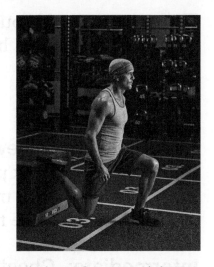
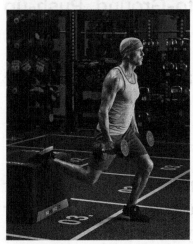

height of your shin to midfoot. (If your knee is on the ground at its base, the top of your midfoot should hook comfortably over its top.) Hook the top of your left foot on top of the box and hop your right foot forward far enough that when you lunge, your front shin stays vertical while your rear knee comes to the ground or close to it.

Advanced: Loaded Split Squat. Lunge as above, carrying a quarter of your body weight in each hand (dumbbells or kettle-bells will work). You can also vary this:

Try carrying half your body weight held to your chest, or load a heavy sandbag on your upper back.

PUSH-UP

Beginner: Chest Elevated (See page 343–344). Start in a plank position and place your knees on the floor, maintaining your tight core and straight line from hips to shoulders.

Intermediate: Chest-to-Ground Push-up (See page 344).

Advanced: Feet-Elevated Push-up (See page 345).

JUMPS

Beginner: Jumping Jacks. Stand with your hands at your sides. Jump your feet wider than your hips, raising your hands overhead, keeping your arms as straight as possible. Clap at the top and jump your feet closed, arms coming to your sides.

Intermediate: Jump Ropes. Keeping your core tight and your elbows in at your sides and your hands turned out, bounce about an inch or two off ground with your knees bent slightly. Spin the rope under using your wrists to drive the action not your arms. Only do one bounce per spin!

Advanced: Double Unders. Increase the speed of your wrist spin to pass the rope under your feet two times per bounce. At first, a slightly higher bounce will help, but with experience this won't be necessary.

For Double Unders, make sure to initiate both spins while the rope is out in front of you. Keep the legs straight. The three most common mistakes are the following:

1. Bending the knees (the rope will catch on your knees).
2. Initiating the wrist spin after the rope is under your feet.
3. Seeing this as having two separate spins. You have to spin it two times now; really whip those wrists around!

Seven-minute AMRAP workout: Do as many rounds as possible of three exercises in seven minutes. Rest for five minutes. Repeat (do a second seven-minute round).

Beginner	Intermediate	Advanced
Down Dog to Up Dog x 5	Feet on Box Push to L x 5	Handstand Wall Walk-up x 2
High Body Row x 5	Low Body Row x 5	Elevated Feet Body Row x 5
Jumping Jacks x 40	Jump Rope x 40*	Double Under x 40*

*If you don't have a jump rope, you can substitute a fast-paced run, bike, or row for 20 seconds.

DOG, L-PUSH, HANDSTAND SERIES

Beginner: Downward Dog to Upward Dog. From tabletop position with your hands under your shoulders and your knees under your hips, press up into an inverted V, pressing your palms into the floor and pushing your hips away. Shift

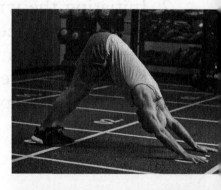

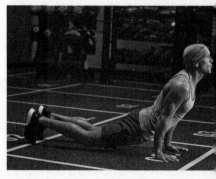

356

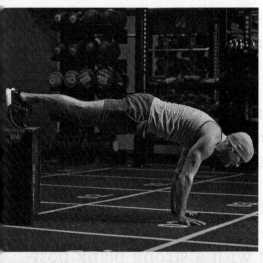

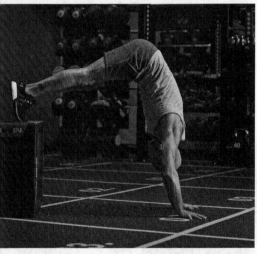

your weight into your hands as you scoop your chest between them, coming into Upward Dog with toes tucked. Lift your hips up and press your chest back into Downward Dog.

Intermediate: Feet on Box Push to L. Start in a plank position, head facing away from the box and your feet flat against its base. Walk your hands in a few inches so your knees bend, lift one knee off the ground, and put your foot on the box. Tighten your core and place your other foot on the box. Keeping your hands and feet stationary, push your hands into the ground and your butt to the sky, moving your chest inward to the box, then lower your hips and bend your knees.

Repeat five times, then walk your hands back out to a plank position and step your feet off the box.

Advanced: Handstand Wall Walk-Up. Start in a plank position with your feet touching the base of the wall. With a very tight core, start to walk your feet up the wall and walk your hands in as far as you are comfortable. The aim is to come all the way into a nose-to-wall handstand with a strong plank position. Reverse the movement to come down. Walk your hands all the way out to a plank position before taking your feet off the wall.

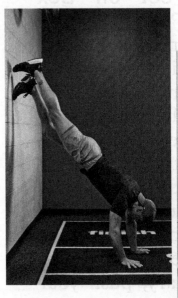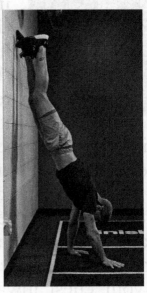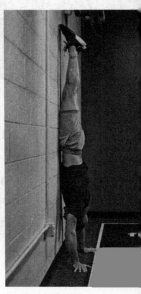

BODY ROW

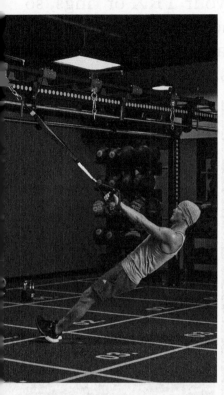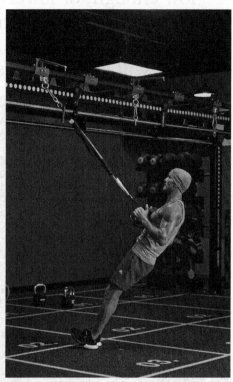

Beginner: High Row. Sit under a chest-high bar and walk your feet out in front of you, legs extended, until the bar is over your upper chest. Grab the bar and lift your hips up, keeping your core and glutes tight and your body in a straight line. You will be at an incline. Starting with straight arms, pull the bar to your chest, squeezing your shoulder blades. Return your body to a straight-arm position. (You can also use a TRX, rings, or even a very sturdy and secure table for this.)

Intermediate: Low Body Row. Use a bar low enough, or lower your TRX or rings, so that your degree of incline is closer to horizontal. A Smith rack at the gym or a sturdy desk will work for this.

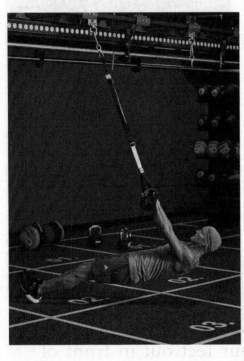

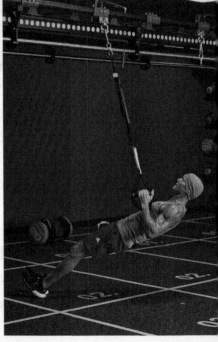

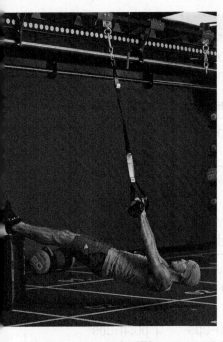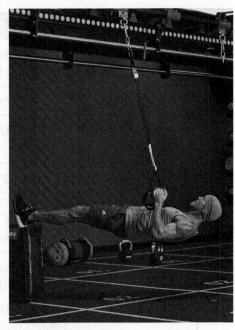

Advanced: Elevated Feet Body Row. From the Low Row position, place your feet on a box so that your body is horizontal. Alternative: Pull-ups.

JUMPS
Beginner: Jumping Jacks (See page 354).

Intermediate: Jump Ropes (See page 354–355).

Advanced: Double Unders (See page 355).

Twenty-minute AMRAP workout. Do as many rounds as possible of three exercises in twenty minutes.

Beginner	Intermediate	Advanced
Battle Ropes x 30 seconds	Battle Ropes x 30 seconds	Battle Ropes x 30 seconds
Farmer's Hold x 20 seconds 1/4 body weight in each hand	Farmer's Hold x 20 seconds 1/3 body weight in each hand	Farmer's Hold x 20 seconds 1/2 body weight in each hand
Bear Crawl to Crab Crawl, 20 steps each way	Bear Crawl to Crab Crawl, 20 steps each way with three push-ups	Bear Crawl to Crab Crawl, 20 steps each way with five push-ups

BATTLE ROPES

Hold one rope in each hand, with a slight amount of slack so ropes drape on ground,

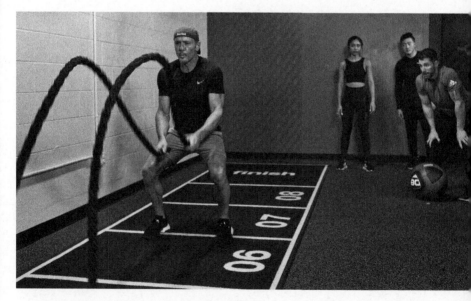

and stand with feet about hip-width apart. Keep your back straight, and raise and lower ropes from thigh high to head high, moving as fast as you can to make a wave along the full length of the rope. You can move both ropes in sync or alternate them. As you pick up speed, sit back slightly on your heels.

FARMER'S HOLD

To start in Farmer's Hold, stand with your feet under your hips, bend your knees and pick up a weight in each hand and stand, holding the weights by your sides with your core strong, shoulders back and glutes tight. Dumbbells or kettlebells work fine for this.

BEAR CRAWL TO CRAB CRAWL

Beginner: Start on all fours with your hands directly under your shoulders and your knees under your hips. Press your hips up to come onto your toes with your knees raised off the ground several inches and your arms straight. Keeping your core tight and your back flat, travel forward with your right hand and left foot moving in tandem and landing together, and then your left hand and right foot. Count one step for every time your left hand hits the ground. After twenty steps, transition to a Crab Crawl. From Bear, walk your hands behind you so your hips come up, and you are now looking upward. You are in an upward-facing table with your knees, hips and shoulders in a straight line. Tighten your core. "Walk" backward with your right foot followed by left hand, then your left hand followed by right foot. Count one step for each time your left hand hits the ground.

Intermediate: Do three push-ups before the Crab Crawl.

Advanced: Do five push-ups before the Crab Crawl.

WORKOUT #6

Seven-minute AMRAP workout. Do as many rounds as possible of three exercises in seven minutes. Rest for five minutes. Repeat (do a second seven-minute round).

Beginner	Intermediate	Advanced
Strict Press x 6, 1/8 body weight in each hand	Strict Press x 6, 1/4 body weight in each hand	Strict Press x 6, 1/3 body weight in each hand
Mountain Climbers x 10	Mountain Climbers x 20	Two-Legged Mountain Climbers x 20
Basic Crunch x 20	Crunch + Sit-up x 20	Hollow Rock x 20

STRICT PRESS

Stand with your feet hip-width apart and with one dumbbell on each shoulder, elbows slightly in front of your body, core tight and

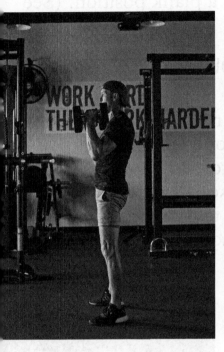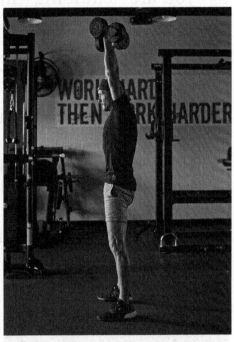

legs static. Push the dumbbells overhead, keeping them in line with your midfoot. Imagine the dumbbells are stationary and you are pushing the ground away with your feet — this will help you stay strong and stable.

MOUNTAIN CLIMBERS

Beginner and Intermediate: Start in a plank position with a tight core. Bring your right knee forward under your chest and land your toes on the ground. Return right foot to plank position as you bring the left knee and foot forward. *Right foot/left foot is one rep.* Pick up a quick pace, almost as if you are "climbing" in a plank position. (See page 320–321.)

TWO-LEGGED MOUNTAIN CLIMBERS

Advanced: From plank position, hop both feet forward under your chest at the same time, then hop back to plank position. Pick up a quick pace and keep your core as tight as you can. Try not to let your hips raise above the plank position.

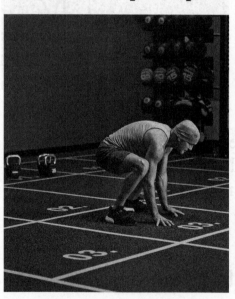
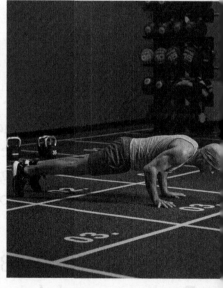

CRUNCHES AND HOLLOW ROCKS

Beginner: Basic Crunch. Lie on your back and bring your feet close in to your butt, arms at your side a half inch off the ground.

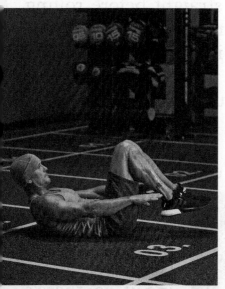

Point your toes like a dancer and lift up your heels. Inhale, then exhale and curl your head, neck, and shoulder blades off the ground, reaching your hands toward your feet. Roll back down.

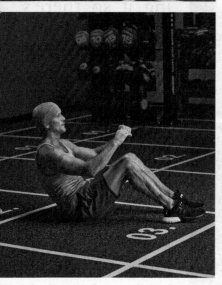

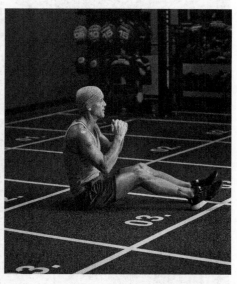

Intermediate: Crunch Plus Sit-up. After your crunch, roll all the way back down to the ground, then do a sit-up, arms still floating at your side, but this time curling all the way up to sitting straight before rolling down to your back. One Crunch + One Sit-up = One rep. If this is hard, you may slide your hands up your thighs. Do not clasp your hands behind your head.

Advanced: Hollow Rock. Lie on your back with your arms extended behind you.

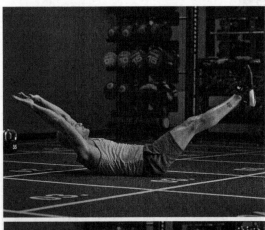
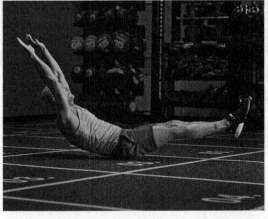

Push your legs together and tighten your core, compressing it so there's no space between your low back and the ground. Raise your arms and legs so you begin to rock on your lower back without moving your shoulders or hips. One rock back and forth is one rep.

In this workout, start with the two 30-second exercises listed in the top box, then immediately start your timer and pick up your weights for the Farmer's Carry and walk as far as you can until you feel you have to put the weights down. Stop the timer when the weights go down, and return to first two exercises. Then start the timer and return to your Farmer's Carry. The workout will be done when your total walk time in the Farmer's Carry adds up to five minutes.

Beginner	Intermediate	Advanced
Jumping Jacks x 30 seconds + Plank x 30 seconds	High Knees x 30 seconds + Elevated Plank x 30 seconds	High Knees x 30 seconds + One-Arm Planks x 30 seconds (each side)
Farmer's Carry, 20 lbs each hand (women); 35 lbs each hand (men), as far as you can walk	Farmer's Carry x 1/4 body weight in each hand, as far as you can walk	Farmer's Carry x 1/2 body weight in each hand, as far as you can walk

JUMPS

Jumping Jacks (See page 354).

HIGH KNEES

Run in place, aiming to get your knees up above your hip creases.

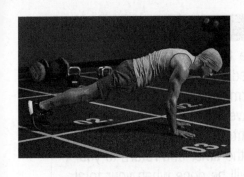

PLANK

Beginner: **Basic Plank.** (See page 348). Lie on your stomach with legs straight behind you, toes pointed toward the ground. Plant your hands underneath your shoulders. Push into your hands and lift your chest off the ground, then lift your knees and midbody so that your entire body, from your heels to your head, is straight, like a "plank," suspended by your toes and hands. Tighten your thigh muscles and pull your belly in and up to engage your core. Imagine a cord pulling your midback upward. Neutralize your neck and place your glance forward, just in front of your hands.

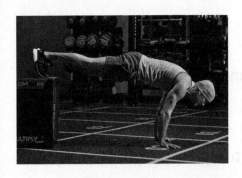

Intermediate: **Elevated Plank.** Start in a plank position, head facing away from the box and your feet flat against the base. Walk your hands in a few inches so your knees bend, lift one knee off the ground and put your foot on the box. Tighten your core and place your other foot on the box. Walk your hands forward so that you form a straight line from head to toe in a plank position with your feet elevated on the box.

Advanced: One-Arm Plank. Start in a strong plank position, your core and glutes tight.

Lift up your right hand and tuck your right arm under your body, reaching across and down toward your left hip. (Imagine trying to put it in your shorts pocket.) Hold for thirty seconds, then return the right hand to the ground and pick up your left.

FARMER'S CARRY

Start in Farmer's Hold, then walk with short steps until you are ready to place your weights down by bending your knees and keeping your back straight. Dumbbells or kettlebells work fine for this.

In this workout, do four rounds of each exercise. For Intermediate and Advanced, follow this formula: Intermediate first round is twenty-five push-ups and a 300-meter row; second round is twenty push-ups and a 300-meter row; and so on. Row as fast as you can, aiming for 90 percent of your maximum perceived effort. You can vary this workout by doing a Sled Push or Bike Sprint instead of a row. (A sled is a weighted apparatus used in functional fitness to push or pull load across distance. Try to run as you push it!) And don't stop between your four rounds. You can rest when it's over!

Beginner	Intermediate	Advanced
Chest-Elevated Push-up x 10	Chest-to-Ground Push-up x 25/20/15/10	Feet-Elevated Push-up x 40/30/20/10
Row 200m	Row 250m/200m/150m/100m	Row 400m/300m/200m/100m

PUSH-UP

Beginner: Chest-Elevated Push-up (See page 343–344.)

Intermediate: Chest-to-Ground Push-up (See page 344.)

Advanced: Feet-Elevated Push-up (See page 345.)

ROW

Start by locking your feet into the straps and grabbing the handle with both hands. Bend

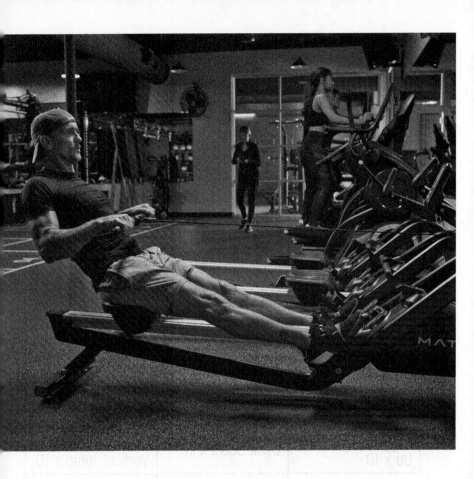

your knees so your body glides to the front of the machine near the handle. Make sure your back is straight. Push into the foot plate and extend your legs. After your legs are extended, use your core to lean back to 45 degrees. Finish by pulling the handle inward until it touches just below your chest. Follow the reverse sequence by extending your arms from your chest, hinge back out of the 45 degrees to upright and bend your knees gliding back to the original position.

Start with four rounds of very short Bike Sprints followed by even shorter rest periods, then take a four-minute break. Then do four rounds of the next two exercises. Once again, a fan bike is preferred.

Beginner	Intermediate	Advanced
Bike Sprints: 10 seconds fast/10 seconds easy x 4	Bike Sprints: 20 seconds fast/10 seconds easy x 4	Bike Sprints: 20 seconds fast/10 seconds easy x 4
4-minute break followed by 4 rounds of:	4-minute break followed by 4 rounds of:	4-minute break followed by 4 rounds of:
Farmer's Carry, 20 lbs each hand (women); 35 lbs each hand (men) x 20 yards	Farmer's Carry, 1/4 body weight each hand x 20 yards	Farmer's Carry, 1/2 body weight each hand x 20 yards
Lie Down Stand Up x 10	Deck Squat x 10	Deck Squat Vertical Jump x 10
Rest 10 seconds	Rest 10 seconds	Rest 10 seconds

BIKE SPRINT

Pedal as hard as you can in timed intervals, then either take it easy (beginner) or rest for ten seconds (intermediate and advanced) as described on the opposite page. After four rounds, take a four-minute break.

FARMER'S CARRY

See page 371.

LIE DOWN STAND UPS

Beginner: Start standing and lower your body to the ground until you are fully prone on your back. You can get down any way you like *as long as you do not cross your feet.* You can squat and bring one hand to the floor or even get onto your knees first for added assistance. Then bring yourself to standing any way you want *without crossing your feet.* If you put your right hand to the floor on the first rep, use your left hand on the second. Again, you can bring yourself to your knees first if it's easier.

Intermediate: Deck Squat. With a mat underneath you, lower into a deep squat. Keeping your hands in front of your chest, lower your butt onto the ground and roll back slightly with your knees tucked to your chest until your hips come off the ground. Using the momentum from that movement, roll powerfully forward, place your feet right under your butt, and stand up, driving your heels into the floor without using hands. You can use a counterbalance to help: Hold a 5- to 10-pound weight to your chest as you go down, then hold it out in front of you like a steering wheel when you stand up so the weight helps pull you forward.

Advanced: Deck Squat with Vertical Jump.
As you stand up, explode vertically, then land in a squat and flow into the next rep if you can.

WORKOUT #10		

Seven-minute AMRAP workout. Do as many rounds as possible of three exercises in seven minutes. Rest for five minutes. Repeat (do a second seven-minute round).

Beginner	Intermediate	Advanced
Handstand Wall Walk-Up x 1	Handstand Wall Walk-Up x 2	Handstand Wall Push-ups x 2
Single-Leg Deadlift x 1/3 body weight, x 5 each side	Single-Leg Deadlift x 1/2 body weight, x 5 each side	Single-Leg Deadlift x 3/4 body weight, x 5 each side
Jumping Jacks x 60	Jump Rope x 60	Double Under x 60

HANDSTAND WALL WALK-UP

Beginner, intermediate: See page 358.

HANDSTAND WALL PUSH-UP

Advanced: Use this variation only if you have mastered a solid handstand with good alignment and core tension. Kick up into your handstand and lower yourself until your head touches the ground or as close to it as possible. Press back up until your arms are at full extension.

SINGLE-LEG DEADLIFT

Hold a dumbbell or kettlebell in both hands. Shift your weight to your right leg and, keeping that knee slightly bent, hinge at the hip, extending your left leg behind you for balance. Lower the kettlebell until your body is parallel to the ground. Driving your right heel into the floor and powering this motion from your hamstrings and glute, return upright.

JUMPS

Beginner: Jumping Jacks (See page 354).

Intermediate: Jump Ropes (See page 354-355).

Advanced: Double Unders (See page 355).

WORKOUT #11

This is a strength workout that will definitely get your metabolism revving. Remember to work at that B-grade level, focusing on form first and foremost, but not moving so slowly that it's easy. If these moves are new to you, practice them slowly at first. You can easily find great demo videos of these online. To keep it simple, we'll use a dumbbell here, but with proper instruction you'll enjoy doing this with kettlebells, too. When in doubt about what weight to use, start with a lighter one and build up.

Beginner	Intermediate	Advanced
Dumbbell Clean and Strict Press x 5 each side Weight: see below	Burpee Clean and Press, 25 lbs each hand (women), 35 lbs each hand (men)	Dumbbell Clean, Press, Front Squat Ladder Weight: See below
	100 reps or 20 minutes (whichever comes first)	60 Double Unders each time you need a break

Beginner: Dumbbell Clean and Strict Press. Choose a weight that you can manage for seven reps maintaining good form before feeling tired. (Experiment first — is this ten pounds? Fifteen? More?) Start with your feet slightly wider than hip-width, dumbbell between your feet. Squat down

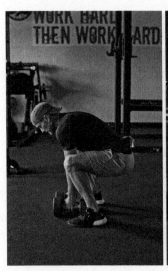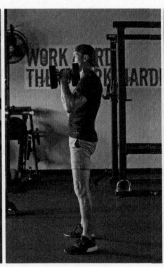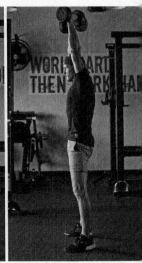

with a straight back and grab the dumbbell with both hands. Pushing your heels into the floor, powerfully drive yourself upward, extending your hips, knees, and ankles and throwing your elbow forward quickly to drive the dumbbell to shoulder height. After you have achieved full extension, receive the weight on your right shoulder. You will end in a standing position. If it's too much weight, you can modify and do one side at a time.

Now perform a Strict Press. Keeping your core tight and your legs static, push the dumbbell overhead, keeping it in line with your midfoot. Imagine the dumbbell is stationary and you are pushing the ground away with your feet — this will help you stay strong and stable. Return the weight to your shoulders, then bend your knees and place the weight back on the ground between your feet. One Clean and one Strict Press is one round.

Intermediate: Burpee Clean and Press. Place both dumbbells between your feet, directly under your shoulders. Squat and place your hands on the dumbbells, hop your feet back to a plank position with a tight core, hop your feet forward, and perform a Clean as described above with both weights simultaneously. From the shoulder position, press the weights overhead in a Strict Press (as described on page 365).

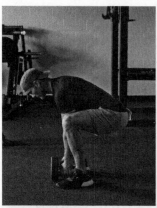 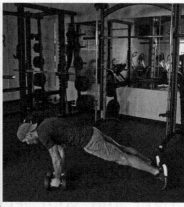 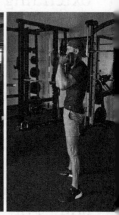

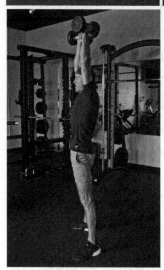

Advanced: Dumbbell Clean, Press, Front Squat. Perform all three exercises in a ladder until your form starts to slip. A ladder is one rep each of a Clean, a Press, and a Front Squat, then two reps of each, then three reps of each, then four reps of each. Each time you need to take a break during the ladder, do sixty Double Unders before you rest. Your choice of weight here: Use the highest weight that you can move with good form for seven reps before getting wonky. Instructions: Clean and Press as above, and from your final Press position, with weights resting on your shoulders, squat as low as you can — hip crease always lower than the knees. Drive the ground away with your heels, and tighten your core as you stand up. Place the dumbbells back on the ground between your feet, stand up, and then start the next rep.

PLAY: LET IT ALL HANG OUT

No matter where you are on your fitness journey, relative newcomer or established athlete, don't forget to let loose on a regular basis. Play is as straightforward as it sounds: At least once a week, be sure to get out and do some kind of movement that is unstructured, goal-free, and (above all) fun. The basic idea? Let out your inner kid and do something that has nothing to do with "getting fit." You're doing it because it feels good. This isn't about being sentimental for childhood. There's a physiological reason for including play as part of your health and fitness routine: It helps you take all the gains you've made in workouts, like strength, power, coordination, balance, and agility, and allows you to put them into practice in surprising ways.

Playing doesn't have to require tons of forethought — it sure didn't when you were young! Start a game of Marco Polo in the

You can take your new workout skills with you everywhere go. I regularly do pool training as part of my regime to keep things fresh, with a mix of water resistance training, martial arts, and cardio training. For a super-simple pool workout, try this:

Stand at the top of the pool and do ten push-ups. Dive in and swim the length of the pool; get out and do ten sit-ups. Dive in and flutter-kick back to start (extend your arms out like a superhero in flight and only use your legs to kick). Repeat ten times. If you're on the beach, you can throw together a workout with minimal thought. Walk lazily for ten minutes to warm up. Then mark a line in the sand about twenty yards out. Sprint as hard as you can to the line, do five push-ups, and do a Bear Crawl back as fast as you can. Take a two-minute break and repeat for ten rounds. Alternate the Bear Crawl with Crab Crawl and spring with speed skips, high-knee skips, and broad jumps. Gather friends and family and make each round into a race.

pool; take a spin at the trampoline gym, go for a family bike ride, or try ice skating for

There are times I'm stuck in a hotel with no access to a gym or even the chance to get my sweat on outside. In those instances, I put together a sequence that I can do in limited floor space and in my regular clothes if necessary. It works just as well when you're at home with your kids — or confined in your office on a deadline.

Do each move five times at a quick clip, and do at least three rounds. The first two are your warm-up/mobility, and the last three take it up a notch.

- Rolling Backbend Prep
- Hindu Push-up
- Full Burpee
- Mountain Climbers (single-leg or two-legged)
- Squat (any variation)

the first time in years. At home with your kids? Get on the floor and explore the world from their point of view, rolling around, lifting them high; or stage a dance-off in the kitchen. It sounds silly — but all these things not only work your body in new ways but also bring instant relief to stress levels. Play is therapy for a nervous system in overdrive.

If you tend to take your health regime seriously, get "un-serious" now and then. Mix it up and have fun! If you and your friends or family have a blast being competitive, add the element of challenge with stuff like who can dive farthest off the diving board, or more organized activities like volleyball, flag football, five-a-side soccer, obstacle racing — you name it. Whatever you pick, the point is to experience moving in all kinds of unexpected ways and directions, to propel yourself through space in multiple ways, to feel what it feels like to launch into surprising bursts of power and hit moments of pure flow and grace. Play — even the really basic recreational kind — lets your mind switch off and lets your body switch on, responding

---

MAVERICK HACKS

On the days when there's way too much coming at you, you can still sneak in your training — here are five strategies to keep your gains up no matter what.

1. Put an inexpensive door-frame pull-up bar at the top of your kitchen door. Every time you walk into kitchen, do five pull-ups. If you're still working on

---

pull-ups, you can either use a rubber-band assist or do negative pull-ups.

2. Each time you walk to the fridge, do seven Chest-to-Ground Push-ups. If you're still working on push-ups, do them with your knees on the ground.

3. If it's game day, switch drinking games for fitness challenges. Each time your team scores, do ten squats, lunges, or push-ups. Each time the opposing team scores, do ten dips or pull-ups. Earn those buffalo wings!

4. On a day when it seems impossible to get dedicated time for a workout, make a totally different goal. If you have great kettlebell form already, pledge to do 300 kettlebell swings during the day, divided into as many sets as you want. (Do this workout for a month, by the way, and you'll see huge gains in strength.)

5. Do chores the old-fashioned way: with lots of gusto and elbow grease. Washing your car or working in the yard all count as moderately aerobic exercise.

and reacting to new stimuli and drawing from the capacities you've been training in your workouts. This helps all the benefits of exercise start to come together.

Mentally and emotionally, you get a super boost when you engage in physical play because it triggers that feel-good blend of endorphins, serotonin, and dopamine. It's also a great way to deepen relationships. When people play together, they get a chance to drop past the facades, shift gears if there's been tension, and relate from an authentic place that is more sensory, less heady. Play lets us be primal together giving us a mechanism for bonding and creating a sense of belonging. So take a minute to look at your week. Amid all the to-dos and shuttling around, taking yourself or a family member here, attending to an urgent need there, where can you claim a pocket of time for play? Schedule it in and stick to it!

SLEEP AND RECOVERY: RESTORING YOURSELF AFTER EFFORT

There's an invisible side to getting fitter and stronger: the necessary downtime that balances all the effort of building things up. It's taken me a few years to get a grip on how important it is to sit back and relax after working out hard; you might think you're

To paraphrase the British movement coach Darryl Edwards, founder of Primal Play, think about exercise like nutrition; it's not just the main meals of the day that matter, it's all the snacks you have, too. Are *they* adding up to a full day of quality food? When it comes to fitness, your healthy snacks are all the ways you move throughout the day. One of the best questions you can ask yourself to keep your body in good shape is: Where can I add movement daily by avoiding doing what's convenient? Act on that two or three times a day, and you're automatically having healthy movement "snacks" that add up to a more mobile, less sedentary life. Some ideas:

Anytime you need to use an elevator or escalator, take the stairs instead. (Or at least part of the way if we're talking about a skyscraper.) Play a game throughout the week: On Monday, I'll walk one floor past my destination, then walk back down. On Tuesday, I'll walk two floors up then down. Wednesday, three floors up then down, and so on.

If you have a short car journey to make, think before you drive. Can I walk or bike?

How many extra minutes do I need — where can I grab that time for that? If you have kids, this is a great way to model a healthy lifestyle for them!

Kicking back with a well-deserved favorite show? Disallow any clicks from the couch. Make yourself walk across the room to whatever device you're watching to press pause, increase the volume, or change the channel. For that matter, why watch from a chair or couch at all? Watch from the floor so you get up and down from ground to standing several times, and stretch and move a little as you go.

doing nothing, but it's *after* the workout that so many of the gains are made. Muscles remodel themselves and, if you've been challenging them with weights and taking in good nutrition, they do their "growing" after you've stopped moving. That's one reason why getting adequate sleep is so important for health and fitness goals. Sleep is when your body goes into self-repair mode and secretes the growth-factor proteins that help you build new muscle. It's kind of like taking a cake out of the oven — or a steak off the grill — and "letting it rest." Sleep is when the really good stuff happens below the surface, your superhero transformation taking place without you realizing it. Skip getting good sleep, and you're compromising the benefits of your workouts.

Sleep is also critical for maintaining baseline health, regardless of the ways it benefits your fitness practice. Some experts suggest it's as important as diet. When you sleep, your immune system has a chance to clean up loose ends, so to speak, protecting you against disease; it's when your brain clears out debris that accumulates all day, too, reducing the inflammation that can cause degeneration as you age, and keeping brain function healthy for longer. Enough quality sleep also helps to regulate your appetite, and research now shows it plays a major role in helping your body regulate a healthy weight. Plus, it restores the energy systems that get drained by stress, causing you to tip into reactive responses.

For that reason, sleep has become more revered in our home than it ever used to be, especially back in my candle-burning years. As an athlete, it's my number one recovery strategy. I try to get enough of it every night, and I admit I fail fairly frequently — learning proper sleep hygiene is my current health homework, and the challenge that I'm trying to turn my discipline toward daily. I struggle with it — primarily because so many ideas and concerns hit my brain when the house powers down and everything goes quiet that it's a true mental practice to stop trying, stop solving, and stop worrying. Secondarily, I'm as tempted as anyone else to watch season this or that of something gripping, and the stack of books I want to get through stands precariously high on the nightstand, calling at me to dive in. But my body's smarter than I am: It's usually tired and ready to power down after what I put it through physically. I'm working on letting my mind follow its lead.

Recovery for an athlete can look like more than a decent night's sleep, however. Anytime I've been training hard, I've learned to cap my toughest workouts to four to five maximum per week and keep a few tools in my kit to help my nervous system decompress and reset. Otherwise I hard-charge from one day to the next and risk getting "under recovered," a state in which the body goes almost into survival mode because it hasn't had a chance to restore. It can start to pull from your energy reserves (like your adrenal glands) and make you really run down and more likely to get injured or crash.

My primary recovery tools involve water: If I'm somewhere warm or on vacation, I'll do some easy swimming, just active enough to feel like therapy for tired muscles, but not so active I'm "working out." I like to swim between the buoys offshore from our house in the Bahamas, or some days, grab a paddle chair and lazily paddle around the island, listening to music. When I'm on tour — aka in the middle of the play-off season — water recovery gets more hard core. I take ice baths in a big metal horse trough. Ice baths aren't for the faint of heart, and in fact nobody should go from zero to sixty on this therapy; it'll be too shocking to the system. (For beginners, the way in is to turn down the temperature in the shower, get it to warm, then do brief periods of cold.) Cold water "hydrotherapy" does wonders for relieving inflammation, swelling, and sore muscles, as well as boosting energy and focus. After our tour workout, I'll do a ritual: Some time in a dry sauna followed by a few minutes in the frigid horse trough. It feels incredible. It's the most invigorating thing I could do after busting my ass working out. When showtime comes, I literally feel on top of the world. The great thing about this practice is that it also has been shown to boost the immune system and bring on better sleep — both benefits

I've noticed. Once the lights go down, I'm in bed pretty quick, and I sleep better than ever.

Of course, cold water and ice baths probably work better for intensity addicts like me. Don't worry: Recovery practices can include all kinds of things that help you relax and restore yourself in a fairly passive way. And it doesn't necessarily have to come after elite-level workouts. Sometimes your recovery will help you "get back to neutral" as Roger would say after hours stuck in your head working out problems, or after long days with emotionally challenging experiences. Maintaining good health involves attending to every level of stress — physical, mental, and emotional. So no matter whether you've hit the gym hard or not, I suggest asking yourself daily, *How and where do I feel "worked" today?* A recovery practice might be in order.

Yin yoga is another good option that involves passively allowing the body to fall open in tight spots, without any effort and supported by bolsters. Gentle foam rolling, as described in chapter 2, can work as well. If you have access to a float tank, which is a Zen-like sensory deprivation tank filled with buoyancy-promoting salt water, explore how it restores the body and mind. Then there's the obvious: A hot bath when you finally get some quiet time, filled with Epsom salts if your muscles are tight. And if you want to restore physical, mental, and emotional at once, try the world's oldest recovery method: meditation. You can do it at home, at work, in your car, with absolutely zero props or accoutrements. (An app can get you started, but for real results, look into learning in person with a teacher.)

CLEAN UP YOUR SLEEP

There are entire books on the subject of improving your sleep. Most experts agree that seven hours is the bare minimum needed for restorative sleep; eight is better, and if you're working hard on changing your body composition with diet and weight-bearing exercise, you may need more. It's not just about quantity of sleep; it's also quality. In simplest terms, quality sleep comes when you are able to fall asleep fairly quickly (not more than twenty minutes), stay asleep through the night, waking only briefly if at all, and are able to return to sleep soon after. Here is my cheat sheet to getting closer to those goals.

- Make the decision: I'm going to bed at 9:00/10:00/11:00 p.m. (whatever it takes to ensure you get the quantity you need). Factor in some time for drifting off beforehand. Many older healing traditions say getting to sleep by 10:00 p.m. is ideal, because that's when a natural "repair phase" starts in the body. Set an alarm an hour before that to remind you to wind down.

- Finish eating at least three hours before bed, so your digestion isn't cranking at high gear as you try to fall asleep. Don't drink alcohol close to bedtime either; it can wake you up as your body processes it. As for caffeine, keep that long-lasting stimulant to morning hours only.

- Take back your night from digital devices. The blue light from their screens disrupts production of melatonin, the hormone that helps you fall and stay asleep. Experts say even using blue-light-blocking software doesn't temper this light enough to stop the disruption. The main recourse is a tough but necessary one:

Turn your phone, computer, iPad, and, yes, even your LED screen TV off at least two hours before bed, preferably more. But if that's laughable, at least for now, try turning off your internet at night and putting your cell phone on airplane mode if you must keep it on.

- Create a ritual. Wind down in the same way each night to help trigger sleep onset. It's like helping your body find a new groove. A hot bath works for some; cold water actually helps, too, if you can stand it in your shower. Dim the lights early. Keep your room cool, and turn off all lights and electronics. Make your bedroom like a cocoon.

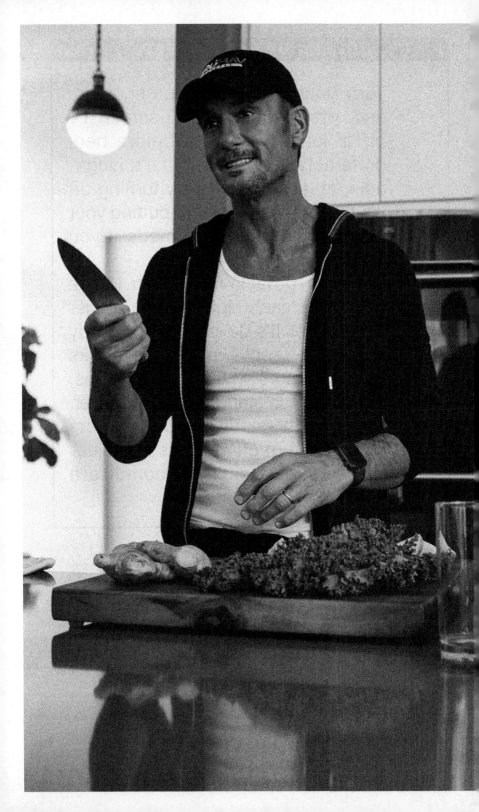

CHAPTER 7

OWN YOUR DIET:
MAKE YOUR RULES

The first thing I like to do when I get a chunk of free time? Go for a swim or take a walk with Faith. The second? Get set up in the kitchen, prep all of the ingredients for something I want to cook, and make us a killer meal.

Working out and enjoying great food aren't at odds around our house. They go together. They have to, because you can't own your health without having both habits, physical exertion and good nutrition, in heavy rotation. A lot of experts suggest that being lean and healthy depends three-quarters on diet and only one-quarter on exercise. While the way you eat obviously influences your body composition, I don't fully agree with that sentiment. I think of it as a fifty-fifty scenario, because a solid workout habit plays a significant role in how your metabolism burns food for fuel and helps flip the switch to a positive lifestyle where you

397

have the energy, clarity, and confidence to make a nutritious eating habits stick. The saying that *does* hold true is that you can't out-train a poor diet. Work out reliably but eat junk or endless sugars and starches, or deprive yourself of quality protein and good fat, and you'll not only function poorly, you likely won't change shape to get closer to the body you want.

I didn't have the greatest food education in the world. The Louisiana I grew up in was all about biscuits, Coke, and mayonnaise eaten off a spoon from the jar, and *organic* was a word they used in California but not so much around our parts. So I had to teach myself how to eat, starting pretty much from scratch. I've seen my share of diet trends come and go, and since I'm a curious person, I've played with a lot of them: low-carb; plant-based; paleo; keto. And what I've discovered is that some of these can be terrific tools to have in my kit for when I want or need them. But for everyday life I take a more baseline approach. I don't want to follow a strict eating plan; I want to eat food! I want it to be as bright, colorful, and lively as possible, but I don't want to get super technical about it. I try not to overdo anything (most of the time). I don't count calories — I eat to fuel my body's needs, and all the vegetables and fiber fills me up each meal so that wondering if I can eat more doesn't really happen. I probably won't ever rigorously count my carbs; I'd rather eyeball that part, having developed a rough idea of what works for me. And I'd rather repeat the same healthy meals frequently than get too caught up in wondering what I can and can't consume. I guess you could say I like to keep my eating as simple as possible.

My approach: Enjoy food that is clean, real, and good *enough.* What I mean by that is that as many of the ingredients I eat as possible come direct from the source (earth, tree, plant, or sea), not a box, bag, or wrapper. That means lots of vegetables and some fruit; protein without any bells and whistles added; and fats that haven't seen an industrial food plant on their way to the bottle, jar, or butter pack. I try to remember that an apple and almonds are as convenient to grab as a snack filled with fake food-like ingredients. And most of the time, my food intake is balanced and wholesome enough to get an unreserved stamp of approval from a nutritionist.

Three to four days a week, I follow a moderately low-carb diet: breakfast is oatmeal with coconut cream and dried fruit or half an English muffin with nut butter and whole milk; lunch is tuna or chicken salad with avocado; and dinner's a great piece of grilled protein, lots of vegetables, some quinoa or half a sweet potato with butter. If I'm training pretty hard, there's a protein shake thrown in midmorning and midafternoon, and full-fat yogurt with unsweetened granola before bed. I haven't gotten so hard core that I eliminate any food that's ever been processed in any form (note the English muffin). It's called doing the best I can within reason and getting to know the impact of all the foods I eat daily. I also have a family I like to eat with — and a wife who's a great cook — so a couple of times a week, it's more comfort than ultra-clean. There might be a pot roast and mashed potatoes in the mix one day, or a homemade pizza with salad on another. But in both cases, they're made from scratch and we know every ingredient that's gone into the pot or oven.

And every now and then, the regimen loosens up to include a chili dog on the road with the guys because we're in L.A. and we have to go to Pink's, and we earned it with our workouts. A cheeseburger *with* the bun, because the kids want to go out after a movie. Or that damn caramel cake that Audrey and I demolished sitting at the kitchen table at Christmas, because we had something to celebrate, and what else can you celebrate with than cake?

I look at it this way: Eating poor-quality food will sneak up on you if you let it, so vigilance is required — now more than ever, when you can easily find yourself eating takeout, snacks, or lattes on a daily basis with zero knowledge of what's actually in them. Yet there's so much information out there about how to eat better, it can easily get overwhelming, to the point where you give up on making a change. I like to keep things simple, and I think most people can stay pretty well on track by implementing five basic food "rules," adapted of course to their personal or ethical eating style, and maybe adopted one at a time so that new habits can gradually sink in and feel solid:

1 Start making your own food, as often as you can. And make it from whole, unprocessed ingredients, with as much organic fare as you can afford, piling vegetables onto your plate or into your bowl next to a palm-size serving of your protein of choice — be that animal protein like meat, chicken, fish, or eggs, or plant-based protein like lentils and beans. If you're a meat eater, try to eat a few fully plant-based meals during the week to

lighten the load and teach yourself to eat plants at every meal.

2 Stay away from empty calories. As a rule, don't drink your carbohydrates — especially not soda and ridiculous coffee-shake concoctions, but also beer and cocktails; if and when you do drink these beverages, make it count — notice every sip, enjoy it, and see if less can be more. When you put together a plate or order a meal, consider every add-on and ask if you really need it. Can you skip the cheese/sour cream/bun/creamy potato salad? Chances are you can. It just takes a second to ask yourself the question. And catch yourself snacking when you're not hungry. Press pause, notice if you're bored/antsy/anxious instead of actually hungry, then try to do something else to fill your time.

3 Eat enough good-quality fats like extra-virgin olive oil, grass-fed butter, avocado oil, unrefined coconut oil, tallow, flaxseed oil, and the naturally occurring fats in foods like eggs, full-fat dairy (if your body likes dairy), fish, meat, and nuts to satiate your hunger. Meanwhile, avoid refined vegetable oils, aka "industrial oils" (mainly canola, peanut, cottonseed, sunflower, soy oils), which are so dangerously inflammatory that a lot of experts suggest they're more deadly than sugar. Most especially steer way clear of food fried in these oils, like French fries, potato chips, tortilla chips, and doughnuts unless it's a real splurge (in which case, bless your food twice, and enjoy it as a treat). It's now known that food fried in vegetable oil is one of the worst things you can put in your body.

4 Keep super-starchy foods like bread, pasta, baked goods, and tortillas for occasional indulgence; their carb load adds up as they quickly turn to sugar in the blood, which makes weight gain more likely. (Many of them contain sugar and often highly processed oils, too.) Other higher-carb foods like whole grains and potatoes can cause similar weight gain for some body types, even beans, legumes, and lentils for some! So, if you're watching your weight or wanting to lose it, try subbing any of these foods for generous portions of leafy and crunchy vegetables or moderate servings of the grain-like seed quinoa instead. This step alone can do wonders.

5 Keep a sharp eye on sugar — not just the kind you add to things, but the grams of sugars listed on the label of any packaged foods or drinks, too. For optimal health, take the ruthless approach: if it's over 5 grams per serving, your blood sugar, your waistline, and probably your mood, too, will thank you for cutting it out.

Maybe you noticed that this list is about two hundred pages shorter than most of the nutrition books out there. What can I say? All I know is that when I follow my five-point formula, I feel good, have lots of energy, don't get hungry or have cravings, and can stay more or less within three days of totally cleaning up my act even with the mashed potatoes I just consumed. I know I can cut down on the comfort foods (especially any bloat-producing wheat and sugar) and go hard on the broccoli to get back to where a camera pointed at me won't make me cringe — at least too much.

And maybe I should add Rule #6. Don't starve yourself! Getting fit, strong, and healthy can't happen from a place of deprivation. Restricting your food intake too much can cause your metabolism to slow down so that instead of feeling and looking

Get familiar with all the foods and drinks you consume daily or weekly. If they come from a package or are bought out on the run, a nutrition label exists, either printed on directly on the package or — very typically — available from the restaurant or retailer. Train your mind to be a detective: How many servings are in the portion size you have? Is it giving you any protein? Are there lots of added sugars? (If you're counting carbs, you can learn how to minus out fiber from the total carbohydrate value to get the "net carb" value.) If it's a processed food and has a lot of fat, it's probably from industrial oils, unless it's a new wave health product — read the ingredients.

better, you get tired and stuck at a place where you physically can't lean out even while eating less food because your body holds desperately onto the fat stores it already has and won't let them go — it gets the message that food is running out and survival is at stake. To get yourself burning more of the fat stored on your body so you lean out, it's better to work out regularly and with some intensity, and to feed your hunger. Build muscle through strength training, because muscle is the engine of your metabolism, and the more of it on your body, the more fuel held in deep storage (i.e., fat stored on your body) you burn. And include some high-intensity workouts that get your metabolism cranking away like a cast-iron stove. When I started getting fit, I had a surprise: To build a leaner, more defined body I had to eat more than I thought, with extra protein to build the new tissues of my muscles and enough carbohydrates to power the faster, harder parts of my workouts. It was kind of a mind-blowing moment to realize that to look leaner and more defined I had to eat regularly and eat enough! The new muscle mass that was developing required significant nutrition; in exchange, this fuel-burning muscle mass helped me lean out more. (Caveat: If you're not looking to build muscle mass, keep protein moderate by following the palm-size rule. Going overboard with protein when your body is not actively in a growth phase can have adverse effects.)

Why not nix the comfort food entirely, you might ask? Because we need good nutrition and we also need to be *nourished*. Faith and I have made family meals a big part of our lives for more than twenty years. They're the anchor of our days with our children, and sitting down to a good meal feeds us not just physically but mentally, emotionally, and spiritually, too. We both believe in eating healthfully, but there has to be a little heart and soul in the whole thing. I'm about as militant as they come about my grilled fish and salad, but nothing gives me joy like making southern chicken and dumplings on the spur of the moment and having my almost-grown daughters run into the kitchen, grinning with delight. Eating right means laying a foundation of physical health, but it's also about connection and sharing and making memories and rituals. We like to "go deep" in our family meals — keep out intrusions as best we can, slow down for an hour, and follow that same workout credo: *Must be present to win.*

Maybe I'm lucky. I've got some wiggle room built in to my genetics; I also work for it, keeping the overall balance pretty dialed in. It may not be the same for you. Everyone's body responds differently to the same kinds of foods, and this depends on all sorts of factors — your body type and how your metabolism is currently functioning; your stage of life and the balance of your hormones (including stress hormones), any food sensitivities you may have, and even the types of bacteria in your gut. My sister says she can't look at a bowl of pasta or it will stick to her; me, not so much. More carbs or fewer of them? Meat or no meat? Dairy-free or milk and cheese friendly? Though many a diet program would love you to believe it, talk to enough people and it becomes clear there's no one-size-fits-all approach to nutrition. When it comes to finding the optimal eating style to make you feel, function, and look your best, your style might be slightly different from my style, and nobody can do the trial and error for you but you.

So how do you know what works for you? Just like paying attention and asking questions can help you tune into the way an exercise session moves the needle on your energy, mood, and strength, so can this basic body awareness deliver volumes of information about your diet. If you're not loving how you're looking or feeling on your current diet, or if the pain of staying the same has gotten worse than the pain of change, it's probably time to try something new. Opt for a full-on whole-foods diet, no processed foods allowed. Or go grain-free or paleo; or make it a basic two-step approach and take out the dairy and wheat. You can even just pick one thing to quit, like sugar, and when that new habit feels solid, pick the next (junky snacks, fast food, etc.). Give each approach a real college try, three weeks at least, always paying attention to (and writing down when you can) how you feel physically, mentally, and even emotionally after your meals. Don't jump ship if you feel cranky at first. Getting rid of foods or drinks you're used to consuming can cause more of an effect than you realize as your body tries to find a new normal.

Frankly, you might try multiple approaches to find your sweet spot — the balance of foods that makes you feel your best, that you enjoy, and that are doable in your lifestyle. Once you land on that spot, don't be surprised if it shifts as your health evolves, as you get older, and as life demands change. Food doesn't exist in isolation. Our bodies are in a relationship with it, and our bodies are constantly changing.

The takeaway? Healthy eating doesn't belong to one kind of expert; it's a journey of getting to know yourself. And pretty much whatever way you want to cut it, healthy eating starts in the same place: cooking food in your kitchen. So grab an apron and show your heaviest pot what you're made of. I've included some of my favorite recipes here — these are the meals I eat often, along with a few splurges. If you're looking

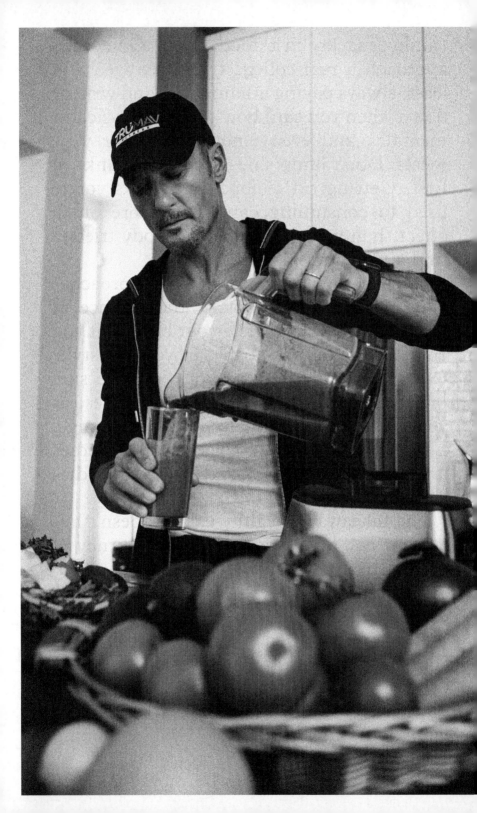

for inspiration, try them out, then adapt them and tweak them to make them your favorites. No matter what you decide to do, simple home-cooked food from real ingredients will make you feel good.

SMOOTHIES

Whether it's whipping up a quick breakfast or getting in a high-protein snack after a tough workout, smoothies are an easy way to get a lot of good things in your body fast. Here are a few of my favorite combinations.

Tropical Smoothie

SERVES 1

1 clementine, peeled
1/4 cup seeded and chopped yellow bell pepper
1 carrot, peeled and chopped
1/2 cup frozen pineapple chunks
1/2 cup frozen mango chunks
1/4 cup frozen coconut chunks*
1 1/2 cups water, coconut water, or unsweetened almond milk

*If you can't find these, use 1/4 cup of shredded unsweetened coconut.

1. Add all the ingredients to a blender and blend until smooth.

2. Add additional water, as needed, to make a sippable smoothie.
3. Serve and enjoy.

Tim's Super Green Smoothie

SERVES 1; DOUBLE IF USING AS A MEAL REPLACEMENT

2 cups stemmed shredded kale, lightly packed
1 apple, cored
Juice of 1/2 lemon
1/4-inch chunk peeled fresh ginger
1 cup water, coconut water, or unsweetened
    almond milk, plus more as needed
1/2 jalapeño, stem removed (optional)
1/4 ripe avocado or 1/2 frozen banana

1. Add all the ingredients to the blender, placing the kale at the bottom — it blends better that way.
2. Blend, adding liquid a little bit at a time, until you reach the desired consistency. This smoothie is naturally high in fiber, so it takes longer to blend than most smoothies — give it time!
3. Serve and enjoy.

Sunshine Smoothie

SERVES 1

1 cup stemmed shredded kale, loosely packed

412

1 cup baby spinach, loosely packed
1 tangerine, peeled
1 blood orange, peeled*
1/3 cup frozen pineapple
1 tablespoon fresh lime juice
1 1/2 cups water, coconut water, or
    unsweetened almond milk

> *If you can't find a blood orange,
> use half a regular orange.

1. Pack all the ingredients in a blender,
   keeping the greens on the bottom.
2. Blend until very smooth, adding liquid
   a little bit at a time, until you reach the
   desired consistency.
3. Serve and enjoy.

Peanut Butter Cup Smoothie

SERVES 1

1/2 banana (fresh or frozen)
1 1/2 tablespoons peanut butter or almond
    butter
1 tablespoon unsweetened cocoa powder
1 1/2 cups skim milk or unsweetened almond
    milk
1/4 teaspoon sea salt
1 teaspoon pure maple syrup (optional)

1. Add all the ingredients except the maple
   syrup to the blender.

2. Blend until smooth, then taste. Add maple syrup if desired.
3. Serve and enjoy.

Berry Blast Smoothie

SERVES 1

1 1/2 cups of your favorite berries (fresh or frozen)*
1 peeled cucumber
1 cup baby spinach
1/2 banana (fresh or frozen)
1 tablespoon fresh lemon juice
1 tablespoon almond butter
1 1/2 cups water, coconut water, or unsweetened almond milk

1. Add all the ingredients to a blender and pulse until well combined; pulsing first helps keep almond butter from clumping up.
2. Add 1 cup of the water and blend until smooth, drizzling in additional water as needed.
3. Serve and enjoy.

BREAKFAST

Eggs and pancakes are a classic pairing, and one that I've long been a fan of, but these days I try to enjoy healthier versions of these simple breakfast foods. By packing a serving of greens into my eggs and a hit of protein into my pancakes, I get the satisfaction of a hearty breakfast without feeling weighed down.

California Greens Frittata

SERVES 4 TO 6

3 whole large eggs
1 cup liquid egg whites*
1/4 cup grated sharp cheddar cheese
    (optional)
1 teaspoon sea salt
1 teaspoon ground black pepper
2 tablespoons extra-virgin olive oil
1 yellow onion, minced
1 jalapeño, minced (optional)
4 cups baby spinach, washed
2 ripe avocados, diced

*If you'd rather separate your own
eggs, use the whites of 6 to 8 large
eggs (depending on size).

1. In a large bowl, whisk together the eggs, egg whites, and cheese, if using. Season with the salt and pepper. Set aside.
2. Preheat the oven to 350°F. Heat a 10-inch, oven-safe skillet on the stovetop over medium-high heat.

415

3. Add the oil to the skillet, along with the onion and jalapeño, if using. Sauté until the onion is translucent.
4. Add the spinach to the skillet — it will look overcrowded at first, but the spinach will wilt down.
5. Cook until the spinach has wilted and the liquid has evaporated. Remove from the heat, and add the egg mixture and avocados, gently folding to incorporate everything evenly.
6. Pop the frittata into the oven and bake for 20 to 30 minutes, or until the eggs have set.
7. Slice and enjoy immediately.

Protein Pancakes, 3 Ways

BASIC PROTEIN PANCAKES

SERVES 4

4 large eggs
4 scoops vanilla protein powder (25 grams protein per scoop)
2 teaspoons baking powder
3/4 cup almond milk or water
Avocado oil spray or butter, for greasing pan

1. In a large bowl, mix the eggs, protein powder, baking powder, and water until a smooth batter forms. It should be slightly

thinner than a typical pancake batter. If the batter seems too runny, add additional protein powder, 1 teaspoon at a time* — this happens because different protein powders are made using different recipes.

2. Proceed to step 3 for plain pancakes, or see the variations below.
3. Melt a small amount of butter in a nonstick skillet or griddle on the stovetop over medium heat, or spray with cooking spray.
4. Using a 1/3-cup measure, pour batter onto skillet. For each pancake use no more than 1/3 cup of the batter — even less will make pancakes that are easier to flip. Cook for 3 to 4 minutes on the first side.
5. When bubbles start to form on the top and all the way around the edges, flip the pancakes, and cook for an additional 2 to 3 minutes on the opposite side.
6. Serve with fresh fruit, a little butter, or a drizzle of honey.

VARIATION 1: LEMON-BLUEBERRY

Ingredients for 1 recipe Basic Protein
    Pancakes (above)
Finely grated zest of 1 large lemon
1 teaspoon fresh lemon juice
1/2 teaspoon almond extract

1 cup blueberries (fresh or frozen; smaller wild blueberries are best)

1. Follow step 1 of Basic Protein Pancakes recipe (above).
2. Add the lemon zest, lemon juice, and almond extract to the batter and whisk until smooth.
3. Melt a small amount of butter in a nonstick skillet or griddle on the stovetop over medium heat, or spray with cooking spray.
4. Using a 1/3-cup measure, pour batter onto skillet. For each pancake use no more than 1/3 cup of the batter — even less will make pancakes that are easier to flip. Cook for 3 to 4 minutes on the first side.
5. When bubbles start to form on the top and all the way around the edges, flip the pancakes, and cook for an additional 2 to 3 minutes on the opposite side.
6. Serve with fresh blueberries.

VARIATION 2: PEANUT BUTTER–BANANA

Ingredients for 1 recipe Basic Protein Pancakes (page 416–417)
4 tablespoons smooth peanut butter or almond butter
2 ripe bananas
1/4 teaspoon ground cinnamon

1. Follow step 1 of Basic Protein Pancakes recipe (page 416–417).
2. Mash one of the bananas with the peanut butter until smooth.
3. Whisk peanut butter–banana mixture into the pancake batter, a little at a time (so a smooth batter is formed).
4. Slice the remaining banana and sprinkle the slices with cinnamon. Set aside.
5. Melt a small amount of butter in a nonstick skillet or griddle on the stovetop over medium heat, or spray the skillet with cooking spray.
6. Using a 1/3 cup measuring cup, pour batter onto skillet. For each pancake use no more than 1/3 cup of batter — even less will make pancakes that are easier to flip.
7. Let the pancakes cook for 1 minute, then sprinkle the reserved bananas on the top.
8. Cook an additional 2 to 3 minutes, or until bubbles start to form in middle and around the edges of the pancakes. Flip and cook an additional 2 to 3 minutes on the opposite side.

LUNCH

When I'm not on the road, I enjoy getting into the kitchen and preparing a lunch I can sit down to. Nothing fancy, just a simple salad or a turkey burger on the grill. Shout-out to our friend Laure at YUM Catering in Nashville, who serves up meals for all of our hometown productions — the kale salad she makes is one of my favorites and was the inspiration for the recipe on page 423–424.

Tim's Tuna Salad

MAKES 1 GENEROUS SERVING OR 2 SANDWICHES

One 5-ounce can white albacore tuna, packed in water, drained
1/2 hard-boiled egg
1/4 cup diced red apple
1 to 2 finely minced fresh red Thai chile peppers (if you like spice)*
1 to 2 tablespoons minced walnuts, toasted
2 tablespoons minced sweet-and-sour pickles (like the bread-and-butter type)
2 tablespoons mayonnaise, plus more if you like an extra-creamy tuna salad
1 teaspoon yellow mustard
1/2 teaspoon sea salt
1/2 teaspoon ground black pepper

*If you're not a spice fan, omit this — or try half a seeded jalapeño to tone down the heat without eliminating it.

1. In a large bowl, gently stir together the tuna, egg, apple, chile, walnuts, and

pickles until well combined.
2. Add the mayo, mustard, salt, and pepper and fold until the ingredients incorporate and the salad comes together.
3. Add additional mayo to reach *your* desired level of creaminess.
4. Serve over salad greens, or as a sandwich. (It's great on an English muffin!)

The McGraw Turkey Burger

MAKES 8 PATTIES

1 pound 93% lean ground turkey
1 pound 100% white meat ground turkey
1 sweet onion, finely minced

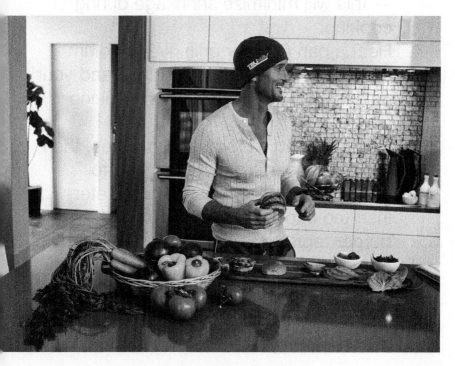

421

1 to 2 jalapeños or fresh Thai chile peppers,
   finely minced
1/4 cup minced fresh cilantro or flat-leaf
   parsley
1 cup shredded carrots
1 1/2 teaspoons smoked paprika
2 tablespoons Dijon mustard
2 teaspoons Worcestershire sauce
Olive or avocado oil cooking spray

1. In a large bowl, mix together all the
   ingredients until well combined.
2. Divide the mixture into 8 equal parts and
   shape into patties.
3. Make a divot in center of each patty
   — this will minimize shrinkage during
   cooking.
4. Heat a pan (or your grill) over medium
   heat. Spray the cooking surface and your
   patties with a light coating of cooking
   spray.
5. Cook the patties for 5 to 7 minutes, then
   flip, and cook for an additional 5 to 7
   minutes, or until a meat thermometer
   inserted into the thickest part of the
   burger registers 165°F.
6. Serve on English muffins, or — if you're
   avoiding carbs — wrap in a lettuce or
   collard green leaf to serve.

Laure's Amazing Kale Salad

MAKES 2 GENEROUS SERVINGS

1 bunch kale (about 6 large leaves, or 1
    pound)
1/2 teaspoon salt, plus more as needed
Juice of 1 lemon
2 tablespoons high-quality extra-virgin olive
    oil
1/2 cup freshly grated Parmesan cheese
    (small crumbles are better than shreds)
1/2 cup raisins
1/4 cup toasted pine nuts
1 teaspoon red pepper flakes
Ground black pepper

1.   First, prepare the kale. Remove the
     ribs, and finely mince the leaves into

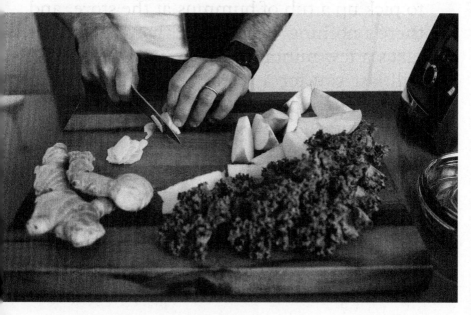

confetti-like pieces. You can do this by hand or by pulsing in a food processor.

2. Transfer to a bowl along with the sea salt, and gently massage with clean hands to tenderize the kale.
3. In a small bowl, whisk together the lemon juice and olive oil. Pour over the kale.
4. Add the cheese and toss to combine.
5. Add the raisins, pine nuts, red pepper flakes, and black pepper and toss to distribute.
6. Taste and adjust the seasoning as needed before serving.

SNACKS

My go-to snack is hummus with some vegetables or gluten-free crackers. Sure, it's easy to pick up a tub of hummus at the store, and there's nothing wrong with that, but it only takes a few minutes to whip up a batch that will last you for a week — and tastes super fresh. There are a million ways you can change up the flavor. I've included a few of my favorites here.

Five-Minute Hummus

SERVES 4 TO 6

1 1/2 cups cooked chickpeas, rinsed and drained (one 15-ounce can is *perfect*)

Juice of 1 large lemon
3 tablespoons tahini
1 small garlic clove, roughly chopped
2 to 3 tablespoons extra-virgin olive oil
1/2 teaspoon smoked paprika
Sea salt
Ground black pepper
Ground cumin

1. Put the chickpeas, lemon juice, tahini, and garlic in the bowl of a food processor fitted with an "s" blade and pulse until smooth. (You can also do this in a high-speed blender.)
2. With the processor running, stream in the olive oil, a little at a time.
3. Add the seasonings to taste and pulse to combine.
4. Serve with sliced veggies for dipping.

VARIATION 1: ROASTED RED PEPPER

Ingredients for 1 recipe Five-Minute Hummus (above)
1 cup diced roasted red pepper, canned or homemade*
1/2 teaspoon sweet paprika
1/4 cup toasted pine nuts

*To roast your own red pepper, simply brush a bell pepper with olive oil and roast in a 400°F oven until the pepper is charred and tender, about 20 minutes. Transfer to a plastic bag and seal. Let steam for 15 minutes, then, using a paper towel, rub the charred skin away. Remove and discard the seeds.

1. Put the chickpeas, lemon juice, tahini, garlic, roasted red pepper, and paprika in the bowl of a food processor fitted with an "s" blade and pulse until smooth. (You can also do this in a high-speed blender.)
2. With the processor running, stream in the olive oil, a little at a time.
3. Add the seasonings to taste and pulse to combine.
4. Top with the toasted pine nuts. Serve with sliced veggies for dipping.

VARIATION 2: CARAMELIZED ONION AND GARLIC

Ingredients for 1 recipe Five-Minute Hummus (page 424–425)
2 tablespoons extra-virgin olive oil
1 medium onion, diced
2 garlic cloves, minced

1. Place a large sauté pan over medium-high heat.
2. Add the oil and onion and cook, stirring frequently, until a nutty brown color, 7 to 10 minutes.

3. Add the garlic, and continue to sauté for a minute or so, or until the garlic is fragrant.
4. Remove the pan from the heat and set aside.
5. Make the basic hummus according to the recipe on page 424–425. Add half the caramelized onion mixture and process until smooth.
6. Top with the remaining onion mixture. Serve with sliced veggies for dipping.

DINNER

There are few things I enjoy more than sitting down to a dinner at the end of the day with my family. On occasion we really go for it and make a celebratory meal, like chicken and dumplings, but mostly we keep it simple, with a healthy protein and plenty of vegetables. I'd rather spend less time in the kitchen, and more time around the table with the people I love.

Chicken Dinner with Quinoa & Veggies

SERVES 4

2 boneless, skinless chicken breasts
1/2 teaspoon sea salt
1/2 teaspoon ground black pepper
1/4 teaspoon garlic powder
1/4 teaspoon sweet paprika

1/4 cup extra-virgin olive oil
Juice and zest of 1 lemon
1 tablespoon pure maple syrup
1 teaspoon Dijon mustard
2 cups broccoli florets
1 cup cauliflower florets
1 cup seeded and chopped red bell pepper

1. 1 yellow onion, chopped
2. Preheat the oven to 400°F. Spray a sheet pan with cooking spray and set aside.
3. Using a sharp knife, carefully slice the chicken breasts in half horizontally, making 2 thinner cutlets from each breast.
4. Slip the chicken into a zip-top plastic bag and pound thin, using the flat side of a meat pounder, a rolling pin, or a spare skillet.
5. In a small bowl, mix together the salt, pepper, garlic powder, and paprika.
6. Season each piece of the chicken with the spice mixture and set aside.
7. In a large bowl, whisk together the olive oil, lemon juice and zest, maple syrup, and mustard.
8. Add all the vegetables to the olive oil mixture and toss until well combined.
9. Transfer the veggie mixture to the prepared sheet pan, making 4 "wells" in the veggie mixture.

10. Add the seasoned chicken to the "wells." Transfer the sheet pan to the preheated oven and cook for 15 minutes.
11. Carefully flip the chicken and return to the oven and cook for an additional 15 to 20 minutes, or until the veggies are cooked through and chicken registers at least 165°F on a cooking thermometer.
12. Serve over quinoa (below).

Simply Cooked Quinoa

SERVES 4

1 cup uncooked quinoa
2 cups water or low-sodium vegetable broth
1 garlic clove, lightly crushed (optional, but adds a nice flavor)

1. Rinse the quinoa in a fine-mesh strainer under cold running water until the water runs clear.
2. Transfer to a pot with a lid, and add the water or broth and the crushed garlic clove, if using. Bring to a boil, uncovered.
3. Reduce the heat to low, cover the pot, and simmer for 15 to 20 minutes, or until the water is absorbed.
4. Remove from the heat and let rest 5 minutes.
5. Remove and discard the garlic clove, fluff the grains with a fork, and serve.

Favorite Fish Dinner

SERVES 4

Four 5- to 6-ounce white fish fillets (such as grouper, swordfish, or halibut)
1 recipe seasoning blend — choose from below
1 recipe salsa — choose from below, or skip, and serve plain
Olive oil cooking spray

1. Season the fillets as instructed in the seasoning blend recipe of choice.
2. Thoroughly oil your favorite skillet with cooking spray, and place over medium-high heat.*
3. Add the fillets to the skillet and cook for 5 to 6 minutes. Flip and cook for 4 to 5 minutes on the opposite side, or until the fish is flaky and a knife inserted into the thickest part of the fish comes out hot.
4. Serve with steamed asparagus and a roasted sweet potato (see page 441–442).

*If you prefer to grill your fish, you can do so on a medium to medium-high heat grill. Make sure the grill and the fish are well oiled. Cook for 5 minutes per side.

SEASONING BLEND 1: LEMON AND HERBS
Finely grated zest and juice of 1 large lemon

2 garlic cloves, minced
1/4 cup minced fresh flat-leaf parsley
1/4 cup minced fresh dill
1/4 cup minced fresh cilantro
1/4 cup extra-virgin olive oil
1 teaspoon sea salt

1. In a bowl or a zip-top bag, combine all the seasoning ingredients.
2. Place the fish in the zip-top bag, and carefully squeeze out all the air.
3. Let marinate for at least 30 minutes, or as long as 2 hours.
4. Remove the fillets from the bag, and pat dry before preparing according to instructions above.

SEASONING BLEND 2: SWEET AND SPICY

1 teaspoon sea salt
1 teaspoon ground black pepper
1 teaspoon coconut sugar*
1 teaspoon garlic powder
1 teaspoon smoked paprika
1/2 teaspoon cayenne pepper
1/2 teaspoon ancho chile powder
1/2 teaspoon ground cumin
Finely grated zest of 1 orange

*You can use brown sugar if you can't find coconut sugar.

1. In a small bowl or zip-top bag, combine all the seasoning ingredients, rubbing the lemon zest into the spices to release the aromatic oils from the zest.
2. Coat the fillets with the spice mixture, and let marinate in the refrigerator for at least 5 minutes, and as long as overnight if you like a stronger flavor.
3. Cook according to the instructions in the main recipe (see page 430).

SALSA 1: TROPICAL FRUIT SALSA

1 1/2 cups finely diced tropical fruit (consider pineapple, mango, papaya, kiwi, or a mix)
1 small white onion, minced

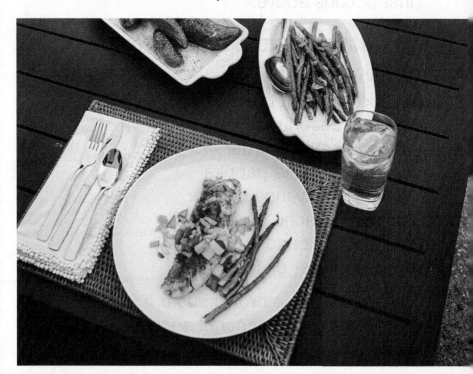

1/4 cup minced fresh cilantro
1 large jalapeño, minced (remove the seeds, if
　　you don't like spice)
Juice of 1/2 orange
Juice of 1 lime
1/2 teaspoon kosher salt
1 tablespoon extra-virgin olive oil

1. Combine all the ingredients in a large
   bowl.
2. Let macerate for at least 10 minutes, then
   serve over fish (or chicken).

SALSA 2: VERACRUZ-STYLE SALSA

2 tablespoons olive oil
1 yellow onion, minced
4 garlic cloves, minced
4 pickled jalapeños, minced (canned or jarred
　　okay)
3 large tomatoes, diced
1/4 cup chopped green olives
1 tablespoon capers
1 tablespoon fresh oregano
Kosher salt

1. Heat the oil in a skillet over medium-high
   heat.
2. Add the onion and sauté until translucent,
   2 to 3 minutes.
3. Add the garlic to the skillet and cook an
   additional minute, or until very soft.

4. Add the jalapeños, tomatoes, and olives, reduce the heat to medium, and cook, stirring occasionally, until the tomatoes release their juices.
5. Add the capers, oregano, and a tiny bit of salt and continue to cook for about 10 minutes.
6. Remove from the heat, taste, and add additional salt to your liking.
7. Serve the salsa over fish, shrimp, or chicken!

Filet of Beef

SERVES 4

Four 6-ounce beef tenderloin filets
1/2 teaspoon kosher salt
1/2 teaspoon ground black pepper
2 tablespoons unsalted butter

1. Season the filets with salt and pepper on both sides.
2. Melt the butter in a large cast-iron skillet* over medium-high heat.
3. Add the seasoned filets to the skillet and cook for 4 to 7 minutes, depending on how you like your steak.
4. Flip and cook for an additional 4 to 7 minutes on the opposite side. Set aside to rest and allow the juices to redistribute.

5. Serve the filets plain, or with the sauce of your choice (recipes follow).
6. This dish is great with a simple baked sweet potato; Perfect Roasted Veggies, such as asparagus (page 441–442); or Garlic Spinach (page 442–443).

If you'd prefer to grill your steaks, brush a grill with oil and preheat it to medium-high heat, then grill the steaks for 4 to 7 minutes per side, depending on how you like your steak cooked.

SPICY CHIMICHURRI SAUCE

1 shallot, finely chopped (or 1/4 red onion)
1 red Fresno chile or fresh Thai chile, minced
3 garlic cloves, minced
1/4 cup red wine vinegar
Juice of 1/2 lemon
1/2 cup finely minced fresh cilantro
1/2 cup finely minced fresh flat-leaf parsley
1/2 teaspoon sea salt
1/4 cup extra-virgin olive oil

1. Combine all the ingredients in a small bowl.
2. Store, covered, in the refrigerator for at least 20 minutes.
3. Serve over steak (page 434–435), or fish (page 430)

RED WINE SAUCE

Reserved pan drippings from the cooked
 steak (above)
1 shallot or 1/4 red onion, finely minced
1 tablespoon minced fresh rosemary
1/2 teaspoon sea salt
1 cup good-quality red wine (something you'd
 drink)
1 teaspoon Dijon mustard

1. Prepare the steak as directed in the main
recipe (page 434–435), reserving the
pan drippings. While the steak is resting,
return the pan with the drippings to the
stovetop.
2. Add the shallot and rosemary and
cook over medium-high heat, stirring
frequently.
3. Add the sea salt and wine and let simmer
until the sauce has reduced by half and
the wine no longer tastes "boozy."
4. Remove the pan from the heat and whisk
in the mustard. Spoon the sauce over the
steak and serve.

Garlicky Grilled Shrimp

SERVES 4

1 pound peeled raw large shrimp, tail on
Finely grated zest and juice of 1 lemon

2 tablespoons extra-virgin olive oil
2 garlic cloves, minced
1/2 teaspoon sea salt
1 tablespoon minced fresh flat-leaf parsley

1. Combine all the ingredients in a large zip-top bag and squeeze out the excess air before sealing.
2. Shake to thoroughly coat the shrimp, then let marinate in refrigerator at least 20 minutes, or up to 2 hours.
3. When you're ready to cook, preheat a grill pan (or your grill) over high heat. If grilling, skewer your shrimp to prevent them from falling through the cracks.*
4. Grill for 2 to 3 minutes per side, or until the shrimp are cooked through.
5. Serve with Laure's Amazing Kale Salad (page 423–424) or Perfect Roasted Veggies (page 441–442) on the side.

*If using wood skewers, soak them in water first, to prevent them from burning. If using round (not flat) skewers, I suggest threading two skewers parallel through the shrimp, to prevent them from spinning on the skewers.

Lightened-Up Chicken 'n' Dumplins

SERVES 8

FOR THE "STEW"

4 tablespoons extra-virgin olive oil
2 large onions, diced
4 large carrots, diced
3 celery stalks, diced
2 garlic cloves, minced
4 boneless, skinless chicken breasts, cut into
  small chunks
1 teaspoon sea salt
1 teaspoon ground black pepper
1 teaspoon sweet paprika
1/2 teaspoon ground sage
1/4 cup whole wheat flour
5 cups low-sodium chicken broth (homemade
  or bone broth is best)
2 cups frozen peas

FOR THE DUMPLINGS

1 1/3 cups whole wheat flour
2 1/4 teaspoons baking soda
1/2 teaspoon sea salt
4 1/2 teaspoons olive oil or avocado oil
3/4 cup skim milk

1. Heat the oil in a large soup pot over
   medium-high heat. Add the onions,

carrots, and celery and stir to combine. Sauté until the onions are translucent and the veggies are tender.

2. Add the garlic, chicken, and seasonings and continue to sauté, stirring frequently, until the chicken is cooked through and the mixture is very fragrant.
3. Add the flour and cook for 2 to 3 minutes, or until the flour is well incorporated. Add the broth and cover the pot. Reduce the heat to low and let simmer.
4. Meanwhile, make the dumplings: Combine all the ingredients in a large bowl and stir to combine, adding more water until needed. A cohesive, slightly stiff dough should form.
5. Shape the dumplings in one of two ways: either between two teaspoons (like drop cookies) for round, fluffy dumplings, or by rolling the dough flat and cutting it into bite-size chunks, for more noodle-like dumplings.
6. Making sure that broth is at a high simmer, add the dumplings to the pot.
7. Cover and cook until the dough is cooked through, about 20 minutes. The dumplings will puff up significantly as they cook. Do not disturb them as they cook, or they will fall apart.
8. At the very end of cooking, add the frozen

peas and cook, stirring now and again, until they are warmed through.

9. Serve and enjoy!

SIDES

Unless it's a holiday or some other type of special celebration (in which case, bring on all the side dishes!), I like to keep my sides pretty simple, clean, and vegetable-focused. I tend to roast or steam whatever vegetables I have on hand and serve them with a simple sauce or just a little olive oil, salt, and pepper. You don't have to know any fancy cooking skills to make a nice plate of vegetables, you just have to get the timing right. The charts that follow will help you do just that.

Easy Steamed Vegetables
SERVES 4

1 pound of your favorite vegetables, cut into bite-size pieces (or 2 pounds leafy greens)
2 tablespoons sea salt
Water
1 large bowl ice water

1. Add the salt and 2 to 3 inches of water to a large pot fitted with a steamer basket.
2. Bring the water to a boil, then add vegetables to the pot. Steam according to the chart below.

440

3. Transfer to the ice water to "shock" the veggies — this will keep them bright, crisp, and vibrant, not mushy.
4. Serve as is, sauté with garlic and olive oil, or drizzle with your favorite sauce.

Vegetable Steaming Chart

Vegetable; cut into bite-size pieces	Cook Time
Sturdy leafy greens (kale, cabbage, collard greens, mustard greens)	4–6 minutes
Root vegetables (carrots, beets, turnips, celery root, sweet potatoes)	10–15 minutes
Snap peas, green beans, asparagus, spinach	3–5 minutes
Broccoli, cauliflower, brussels sprouts, peppers	6–8 minutes

Perfect Roasted Veggies

SERVES 4

1 1/2 pounds of your favorite vegetables, cut into bite-size pieces
4 garlic cloves, thinly sliced
2 tablespoons minced fresh rosemary
1 thinly sliced jalapeño (optional)
1/2 teaspoon sea salt
1/2 teaspoon paprika
1/4 cup extra-virgin olive oil

1. Preheat the oven to 425°F.
2. In a large bowl, combine the garlic, rosemary, jalapeño, if using, salt, paprika, and olive oil.
3. Add the veggies to the garlic-oil mixture and toss to combine.
4. Transfer to a sheet pan and roast until tender on the inside and golden brown on the edges — see chart below for cooking times.
5. Serve and enjoy.

Vegetable Roasting Chart

Vegetable; cut into bite-size pieces	Cook Time
Asparagus, green beans, snap peas, sliced cabbage	10–15 minutes
Broccoli, cauliflower, fennel, brussels sprouts, onions, eggplant, radishes	20–25 minutes
Mushrooms, okra, tomatoes, peppers	15–20 minutes
Sweet potatoes, beets, carrots, turnips, parsnips, potatoes	35–40 minutes

Garlic Spinach

SERVES 4

2 1/2 pounds fresh spinach
2 tablespoons extra-virgin olive oil
2 garlic cloves, thinly sliced
1 jalapeno, thinly sliced (optional)

1/2 teaspoon sea salt

Finely grated zest of 1 lemon

1. Rinse the spinach under cold running water and pat dry. If using regular spinach (not baby spinach), chop it into bite-size pieces. It'll seem like a lot of spinach, but it'll shrink!
2. Heat the olive oil in your largest sauté pan over medium heat.
3. Add the garlic, jalapeño, if using, the salt, and lemon zest. Sauté until the garlic has softened and is very fragrant.
4. Using a slotted spoon, remove the garlic mixture from the pan, leaving the oil. Set the garlic aside for later.
5. Add the spinach to the pan and turn up the heat. Sauté over high heat until the spinach has wilted and all the liquid has evaporated.
6. Return the garlic to the spinach, stir to combine, and serve.

TREATS

I'll admit I have a sweet tooth, and when I'm not aiming to be in my very best performance shape, I indulge in a treat every now and then. Because I'll have a small serving, I like to really make it count — I love rich flavors, and as you can see from these recipes, I definitely love chocolate.

Laure's Sweet & Salty Cookies

MAKES ABOUT 20 COOKIES

1 cup (2 sticks) unsalted butter
2 cups all-purpose flour
1 teaspoon baking soda
3/4 teaspoon kosher salt
1 cup packed dark brown sugar
1/3 cup granulated sugar
2 large eggs, at room temperature
2 teaspoons pure vanilla extract
2 cups crushed thick-cut plain potato chips
1 1/2 cups bittersweet chocolate chips
    (preferably 72% cacao)
Flaky sea salt such as Maldon

1. Cook the butter in a medium saucepan over medium heat, stirring often, until it foams and then browns, 5 to 8 minutes. Pay close attention, as butter goes from nutty and brown to burnt quickly.
2. Scrape the butter into a large bowl and set aside to cool slightly.
3. Meanwhile, whisk the flour, baking soda, and kosher salt in a medium bowl to combine.
4. Add the brown sugar and granulated sugar and the cooled browned butter to the bowl of an electric mixer. Beat on medium speed until incorporated, about 1 minute.

5. Add the eggs and vanilla, increase the mixer speed to medium-high, and beat until the mixture lightens and begins to thicken, about 1 minute.

6. Reduce the mixer speed to low. Add the dry ingredients and beat to combine.

7. Mix in the crushed potato chips and chocolate wafers by hand with a wooden spoon or a rubber spatula.

8. Let the dough sit at room temperature at least 30 minutes to allow the flour to hydrate. The dough will look very loose at first, but will thicken as it sits.

9. Place a rack in middle of the oven and preheat to 375°F. Line two cookie sheets with parchment paper.

10. Using a 1/2-ounce ice cream scoop or two tablespoons, portion out 10 balls of

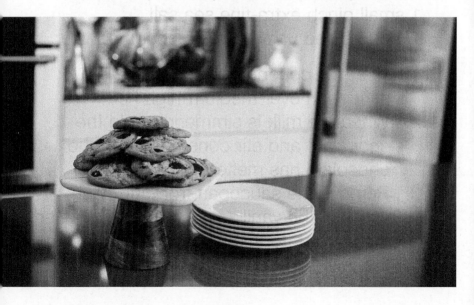

the dough per baking sheet, spacing them about 3 inches apart. (You can also form dough into ping-pong–size balls with your hands.) Do not flatten the dough ball or overcrowd the cookie sheets; the cookies will spread as they bake.

11. Sprinkle each cookie with sea salt.
12. Bake until edges of the cookies are golden brown and firm but the centers are still soft, 9 to 11 minutes.

Dark Chocolate Truffles

MAKES 9 TO 15 TRUFFLES

1/2 cup full-fat coconut milk or heavy cream
9 ounces chopped bittersweet chocolate
    (bittersweet chocolate chips will work also)
1 tablespoon pure vanilla extract
1 small pinch extra-fine sea salt
1/4 cup sifted unsweetened cocoa powder

1. Heat the coconut milk or cream in a saucepan over medium-high heat.
2. When the milk is simmering, add the chocolate and stir constantly until the chocolate has melted.
3. Remove the saucepan from the heat, whisk in the vanilla and sea salt. Transfer the mixture to a shallow, refrigerator-friendly dish.

4. Let cool until set; 2 to 3 hours in the refrigerator.
5. Using a tablespoon-size scoop or two tablespoons, scoop out truffle-size portions of the mixture and place on a plate. The truffles won't be perfect at this point*
6. Quickly roll each portion between your hands into a round truffle (wear rubber gloves if you don't want to get messy).
7. When all the truffles are formed, toss them in cocoa powder to coat.
8. Serve immediately, or store in the refrigerator for 3 to 4 days. Let come to room temperature before serving. You can also freeze the truffles for up to 3 months.

*You can chop your truffle mixture into cubes, if you'd prefer square-shaped truffles — your call.

Healthier Chocolate Cake

MAKES ONE 8-INCH SINGLE-LAYER CAKE

4 ounces bittersweet chocolate chips (approximately 1/3 cup)
1/4 cup (1/2 stick) unsalted butter
1/4 cup unsweetened pure pumpkin puree*
1/4 cup unsweetened cocoa powder
1 teaspoon pure vanilla extract

1/4 teaspoon sea salt
3/4 cup honey
3 large eggs
Flaky sea salt, for sprinkling

*You can also use mashed sweet potato or unsweetened applesauce.

1. Preheat the oven to 375°F. Spray an 8-inch springform pan generously with oil and set aside.*
2. In a small pot over very low heat, melt together the chocolate and butter, stirring frequently until completely smooth. (You can also do this in the microwave in 30-second intervals.)
3. In large bowl, combine the pumpkin puree, cocoa powder, vanilla, sea salt, and honey.
4. Add the melted chocolate and whisk until cooled to room temperature.
5. Add the eggs and whisk until completely smooth and a little fluffy, 3 to 4 minutes by hand (or a minute in a stand mixer).
6. Pour the batter into the prepared pan and smooth the top with a spatula. Sprinkle with sea salt.
7. Bake the cake until the center looks firm or until a toothpick inserted in the center comes out clean, about 25 minutes.
8. Allow the cake to cool in the pan for at

least 15 minutes before removing from pan. Chill before serving.

*If you don't have a springform pan, use a silicone cake pan, or line the bottom and sides of a regular cake pan with parchment paper.

A TRUMAV shows up every day, focuses on the goal, defies the odds, encourages others, puts in the time, works hard, then works harder, overcomes obstacles, envisions the future, embraces the grind, believes everyone is worthy of a healthy life, dreams big, answers to something greater, remains resilient despite challenges, shows courage in the face of adversity, works hard for results, trusts we are stronger together, gives their all.

CONCLUSION

NEVER STOP MOVING

I've been lucky. I've seen music heal people and inspire them; I've sung songs that make grown men cry and cause couples to stare into each other's eyes, swept away in the feelings that brought them together. No matter which side of the stage you're on, there's nothing like music to let you drop your worries and remember what matters most: love, joy, and connection. But when that moment of suspended reality stops and real life starts back up, it can feel a lot harder. Have you ever noticed how the things that bring you the greatest joy, like your kids, your relationships, your job — or some days your whole life — can also bring you the most stress? There's only so much you can control, and the rest of it is racing by faster and faster, year after year. It'll all become a whirlwind if you let it. So, in closing, let me remind you of the most important reason for this book: you.

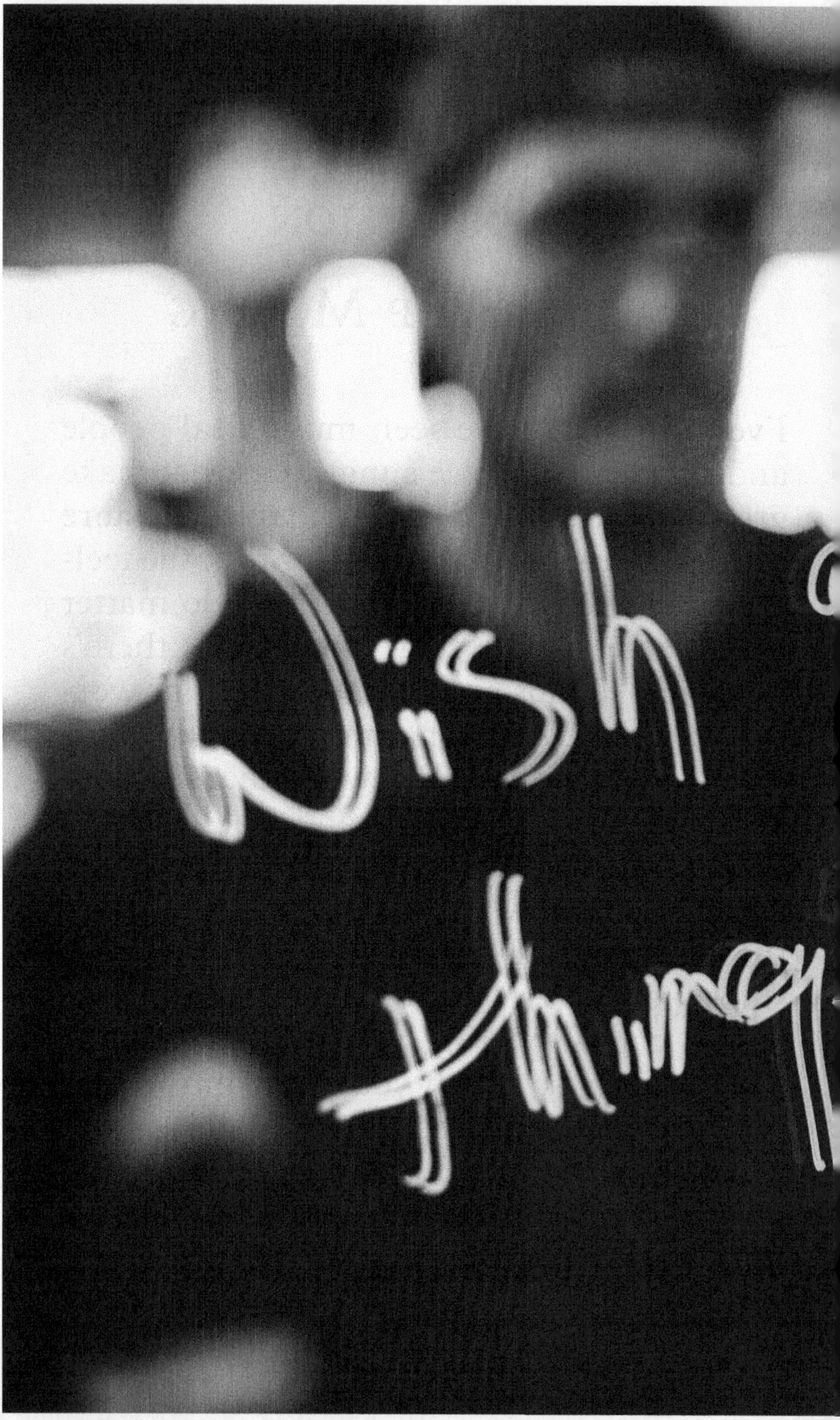
Wish

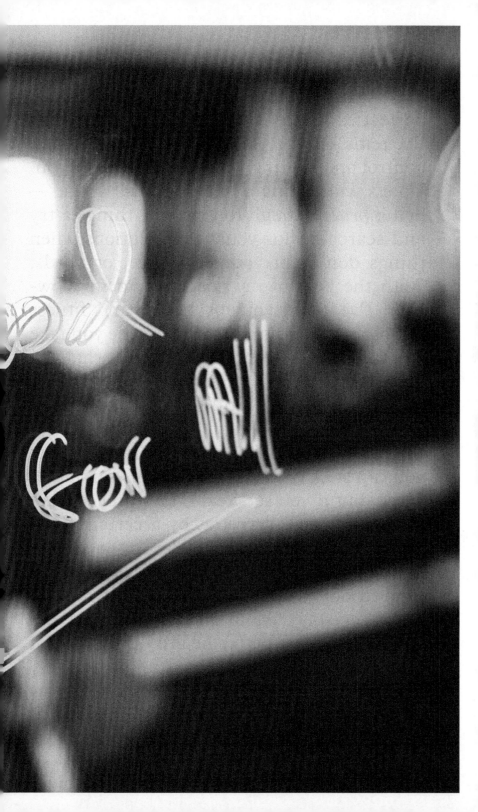

Only you can take the journey toward your best health and life. That doesn't mean you have to master all of it or create a totally perfect existence. But it does require taking the reins on the pieces of life that you can control and finding what works best for you. That's what being a maverick's all about — being brave enough to give new things a try and searching for your own solutions when things don't suit your body, life, or needs. With the help of my coaches and my cowriter, I've given you my health and fitness philosophy as it stands today. I hope you take the pieces that work for you and whatever isn't a fit — let it go. You won't hurt my feelings! We're all different! But grab on to what works for you and then keep searching for the right balance, the mix of practices that you can stick with and enjoy. This can take a while, but if you see health as a process, not a destination to arrive at by a certain date, you'll always be on track. Here's the God's-honest truth: I never feel like I've got it all figured out or that I've arrived anywhere. I just try to stay curious and keep moving and evolving toward better health — not that it always feels easy.

Every journey has high points and low points and lots of grunt time making it through the flats. Some days will seem harder than others. Other days, or weeks, you might lose the way entirely, like a storm caught you, turned you around, and made the path seem impossible to find. If you're anything like me, you'll fail miserably at points, and even your best efforts to succeed will totally falter for a while. But I say, stick with it and try to accept it all, the peaks *and* the valleys. Remember your Whys, connect to your drive, then move again tomorrow. Because if there's one thing I've learned, it's that the longer I commit to this lifestyle, the better I get at finding the road again after those storms hit. I still get lost, but I do get back on track a little quicker than I used to. That's progress and I'll take it!

You likely got the message by now that I believe community is the glue that holds this all together. So, as you set off on your own trip, ask yourself two simple questions: Who do you support? And who supports you, to be as healthy as you can be? Maybe you can't think of anyone at first — that's okay. Just like the right diet or exercise, community can take some time and effort to find. But you can find it, or build it if you need. And it may include people you haven't met yet. Even if your family is your number one reason and motivation to be healthy, bear in mind that your fitness community may include others. Find the folks who will show up to work out alongside you or set shared goals with you, even from afar. Support, accountability, and the occasional tough talk from someone who's sweating alongside you will do wonders.

Even with a motivational crew at your back, ultimately only you can do the work, and for that you have to believe you're worth the effort. Really believe it! If you can't get there fully at first, cut yourself some slack. Feeling worthy doesn't always come naturally. Sometimes you'll get a rush of self-worth that inspires you to hurdle buildings and smash your personal bests, but other times you gotta fake it till you make it. When you hit a slump, go back to the old put-your-own-oxygen-mask-on-first idea. You want to be there fully awake and capable to take care of the people, the animals, and the land or places in nature that need you to be on your game. That can't happen if your health is flailing and you've got nothing to give. If you can't believe in yourself for yourself, believe in yourself for others. That's my trick for the down days: I remember how much I want to be here for my wife, my girls, my family, my friends, my team on and off the road, and my fans. That reminds me: I want an amazing, vibrant life for myself. I know you have that hunger in you, too — you must have, if you've picked up this book in the first place!

So move your body today and move again tomorrow. Remember to breathe and release whatever's in the way of feeling good. Be humble enough to listen to your body while you ask it to perform for you. And always remember to be kind to yourself, even while you test yourself. You're on the path to owning your health. You've already made it so far. Give yourself a fist bump if you have to — or give one to someone else and get one in return. Good luck. Don't give up. And let me know how it goes!

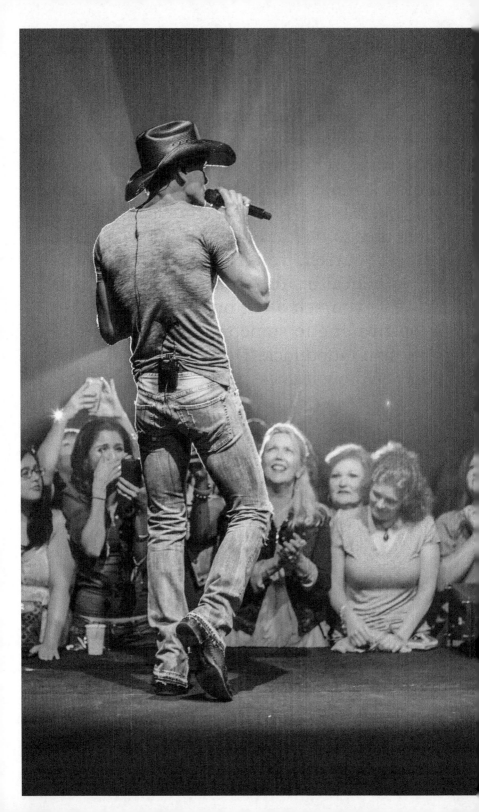

ACKNOWLEDGMENTS

About three years ago, Tim Ferris wrote a book called *Tribe of Mentors*. He graciously included me in the book by asking me to answer a few questions about focus and life-changing habits. All of my answers lead back to exercise and fitness. In fact, my team and I realized that I could talk for hours about how much my fitness routine had changed my outlook on discipline and health. So I have to first say thank you to Mr. Ferris, for asking some great questions.

Thanks to my co-writer, Amely Greeven, for bringing her unique knowledge and point of view to the book, along with so much thought and care. Thank you to Roger Yuan who has shaped my fitness attitude and workout plan over the past seven years more than anyone else. I speak about Roger often in the book, but it's impossible to quantify the mark his knowledge and spirit have made on me and my thinking, not to mention my physical body. Thanks to my band — Adam, Billy, Bobby, Dave, Dean, Denny, and especially EJ, Kevin, Papa, Billy, Deano, and Denny — for taking the time to interview with us. Thanks to everyone on my team, on and off the road. You push me to be my best by always bringing your best. Special thanks to Kelly Clague and Scott Siman for your belief in this book and for helping bring it to life.

Thank you to Julie Will and the team at HarperWave for your partnership and guidance; to Cait Hoyt at CAA for your passion in getting this book to happen; to Coach Mario Cocco and Coach Adam Ticknor for your help with the drills and photoshoot. To my friend Peter Taunton and all of the good people at SNAP Fitness and my TRUMAV Fitness friends and partners, Wirth and Vic Campbell. And to Kate Holzhauer for help getting our recipes into shape.

It is so important to have the Why's that drive you. So in closing, my biggest thanks to my Reasons for waking up each day: my girls — Faith, Gracie, Maggie, and Audrey. Without them anchoring me and supporting me, I would have no transformation story to tell. And thanks to my mom, who raised us by showing us a firsthand example of strength and hard work in action. Thank

460

you to my family, my sister Sandy for her inspiring story to add to the book, as well as my sisters Tracey and Cari; and my brothers, Mark and Matthew. I'd be remiss to not thank my uncle Hank and my father, Tug, for letting me see the fearlessness and tenacity that come with being a professional athlete. "Ya Gotta Believe."

Finally, I'd like to dedicate this book to my high school coach, Larry "Lub" Butler. You never know how much you can change one child's life for the better by simply showing up consistently. Coach Butler encouraged me to work hard on and off the field, to bring personal and athletic integrity to every game, and to be part of a community by being responsible to my teammates through the right attitude and work ethic. He helped shape my athletic ability and helped form the foundation of who I am as a person today. Hopefully, my sharing my story in this book will carry on his example and inspire others.

Thank you so much for reading.

Tim

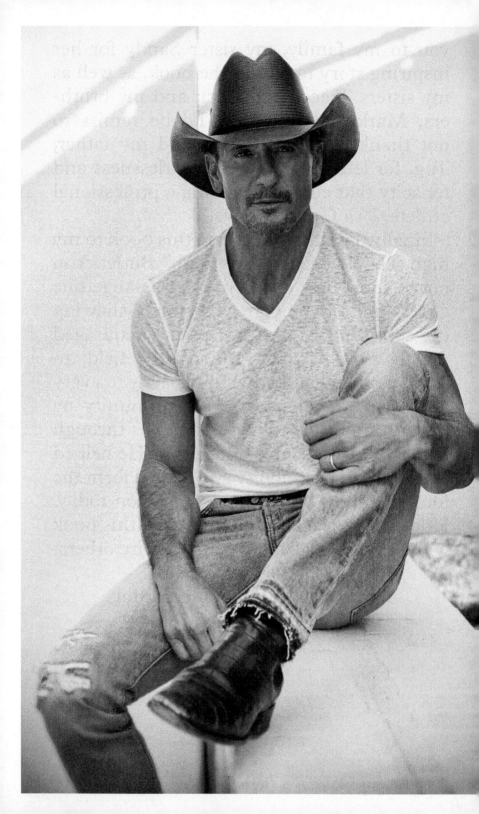

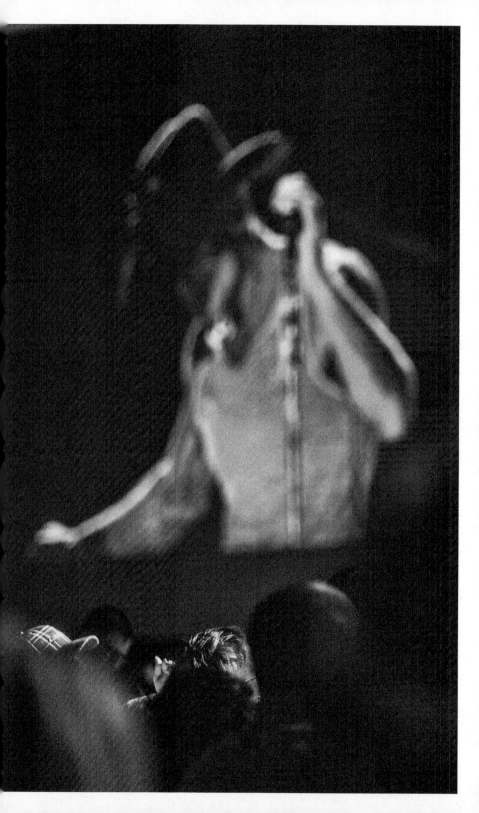

INDEX

476

486

ABOUT THE AUTHOR

Tim McGraw is a Grammy Award–winning entertainer, author, and actor who has sold more than fifty million records worldwide and has dominated the charts with forty-three number one singles. He is the most-played country artist since his debut in 1992, has three *New York Times* bestselling books to his credit, and has acted in such movies as *Friday Night Lights* and *The Blind Side*. He is the founder and inspiration behind the health-and-fitness brand TRUMAV. McGraw is considered one of the most successful touring acts in the history of country music. His last solo project spawned one of the biggest hit singles of all time, "Humble and Kind," whose message continues to impact fans around the world.

The employees of Thorndike Press hope you have enjoyed this Large Print book. All our Thorndike, Wheeler, and Kennebec Large Print titles are designed for easy reading, and all our books are made to last. Other Thorndike Press Large Print books are available at your library, through selected bookstores, or directly from us.

For information about titles, please call:
(800) 223-1244

or visit our website at:
http://gale.cengage.com/thorndike

To share your comments, please write:
Publisher
Thorndike Press
10 Water St., Suite 310
Waterville, ME 04901